Cancer Chemotherapy Care Plans Handbook

THIRD EDITION

Margaret Barton-Burke, RN, PhD (c)
Principal, Oncology Consulting Services
Boston, Massachusetts

Gail M. Wilkes, RN, MS, AOCN
Oncology Nurse Practitioner/Coordinator Breast Oncology
Gillette Center for Women's Cancers
Massachusetts General Hospital
Boston, Massachusetts

Karen C. Ingwersen, RN, MSN, OCN
Clinical Nurse IV
Beth Israel Hospital
Boston, Massachusetts

D0151904

JONES AND BARTLETT PUBLISHERS
Sudbury, Massachusetts
BOSTON   TORONTO   LONDON   SINGAPORE

6/2502

World Headquarters
Jones and Bartlett Publishers
40 Tall Pine Drive
Sudbury, MA 01776
978-443-5000
info@jbpub.com

Jones and Bartlett Publishers Canada
2406 Nikanna Road
Mississauga, ON L5C 2W6
Canada

Jones and Bartlett Publishers International
Barb House, Barb Mews
London W6 7PA
UK

The selection and dosage of drugs presented in this book are in accord with standards accepted at the time of publication. The authors, editors, and publisher have made every effort to provide accurate information. However, research, clinical practice, and government regulations often change the accepted standards in this field. Before administering any drug, the reader is advised to check the manufacturer's product information sheet for the most up-to-date recommendations on dosage, precautions, and contraindications. This is especially important in the case of drugs that are new or seldom used.

Library of Congress Cataloging-in-Publication Data
Barton-Burke, Margaret.
   Cancer chemotherapy care plans handbook / Margaret
Barton-Burke, Gail M. Wilkes, Karen C. Ingwersen.—3rd ed.
   p. cm.
Includes bibliographical references.
ISBN 0-7637-1481-X
1. Cancer—Chemotherapy—Handbooks, manuals, etc. 2.
Cancer—Nursing—Handbooks, manuals, etc. 3. Nursing care
plans—Handbooks, manuals, etc. 4. Antineoplastic
agents—Handbooks, manuals, etc. I. Wilkes, Gail M. II.
Ingwersen, Karen. III. Title.
   RC271.C5 B87 2002
   610.73'698—dc21

2001038541

Production Credits
Acquisitions Editor: Penny M. Glynn
Associate Editor: Thomas Prindle
Production Editor: Jon Workman
Manufacturing Buyer: Amy Duddridge
Marketing Manager: Taryn Wahlquist
Editorial Production Services: Carlisle Publishers Services
Typesetting: Carlisle Publishers Services
Cover Design: Philip Regan
Printing and Binding: Malloy Lithographing
Cover Printing: Malloy Lithographing

Printed in the United States of America

05   04   03   02   01   10   9   8   7   6   5   4   3   2   1

Contents

SECTION II Most Commonly Used Cancer Chemotherapeutic Drugs with Accompanying Care Plans 135

APPENDICES

Appendix 1   Chemotherapy Checklist and Nursing
Guidelines   468

Appendix 2   Extravasation   485

Preface

Two books, *Cancer Chemotherapy: A Nursing Process Approach* and *Cancer Chemotherapy Care Plans*, are companion textbooks that were written to assist cancer nurses to give quality care to individuals with cancer who are receiving chemotherapy. Ten years later these editions endure and can be used by both novice and experienced nurses. *Cancer Chemotherapy Care Plans* is a pocket edition—an abbreviated version of the larger book. Only the most commonly used cancer chemotherapeutic agents are included in this latest edition of the handbook. All side effect information is contained in easy-to-read tables and appendices. The book is intended to be practical, comfortable, and in an easy-to-use size, especially in clinical situations. For additional information on chemotherapeutic agents not found in this book or less frequently used chemotherapeutic agents, the reader is referred to *Cancer Chemotherapy: A Nursing Process Approach* by Barton-Burke, Wilkes, and Ingwersen.

The nursing process is the basis for nurses' scope of practice. Nursing diagnosis is an integral part of the nursing process. This book and the larger edition integrate the nursing process, including nursing diagnosis, with the administration of cancer chemotherapeutic agents. The information included in this handbook is important for the safe administration of these medications.

For over ten years, the field of oncology nursing and cancer chemotherapy drug development has changed and is changing dramatically in ways never dreamed of before. The number and type of chemotherapeutic agents are increasing in unprecedented numbers and nurses using this text are cautioned to be informed when administering cancer chemotherapy. This book is not meant to replace any hospital formulary or manufacturer information. The authors and publisher of this book have made every effort to ensure that the dosage regimens set forth in the text are accurate and in accord with current labeling guidelines at the time of publication. However, in view of the constant flow of information resulting from ongoing research and clinical experience as well as changes in government regulations, nurses are urged to check the package insert of each drug they plan to administer to be certain that changes have not been made in its indications or contraindications or in the recommended dosage for each use. This is particularly important when a drug is new or infrequently employed.

Acknowledgments

We wish to acknowledge the people with cancer for whom we have cared and their family members. They have taught us a great deal about cancer and nursing and about life.

We also thank our respective families, for without their love, support, and encouragement projects such as this would not come to fulfillment. Our families make all the hard work worthwhile.

Margaret Barton-Burke

Gail M. Wilkes

Karen C. Ingwersen

Section I

Toxicities of Chemotherapy

OVERVIEW

Chemotherapeutic agents damage proliferating and resting cells, healthy and cancerous cells alike. The most vulnerable cells are those with rapid doubling times in the hematopoietic, integumentary, gastrointestinal, respiratory, cardiovascular, genitourinary, nervous, and reproductive systems. This portion of the book offers recommended nursing care for patients receiving cancer chemotherapy based on the National Cancer Institute's (NCI) Common Toxicity Criteria (Table 1) and follows an outline format. This section highlights potential problems or nursing diagnoses and the assessment parameters, as well as the drug and dose-limiting side effects for chemotherapeutic agents. This foundation forms the design for nursing care of the cancer patient receiving chemotherapy.

The organization of this section relates to Table 1; subsequent tables offer expanded and detailed information regarding NCI toxicities and the nursing care involved with these specific side effects. For example, the nursing care involved with the toxicities of the blood and bone marrow can be found in Table 2. Nursing care for the gastrointestinal toxicities can be found in Tables 3–5. Another category of toxicities according to NCI criteria affects the liver, and care notes can be found in Table 6.

Table 7 is entitled "Relative Risks of Chemotherapeutic Agents: Nephrotoxicity," Table 8 is a standardized care plan for the patient experiencing alopecia, and Table 9 offers a care plan for the patient experiencing sexual dysfunction. Although seen less frequently, pulmonary and cardiac toxicities can be observed in several chemotherapeutic agents, and information regarding these agents can be found in Tables 10 and 11, respectively. For patients with changes in blood pressure there is no specific nursing care other than that which would normally be given to patients with either hypertension or hypotension. However, neurotoxicity can be seen with several chemotherapeutic agents, especially in high-dose protocols; therefore, Table 12 offers a standardized care plan for the patient experiencing neuropathy. Specific information related to skin and allergic reactions can be found in Appendices 2 and 3. Finally Table 13 offers a nursing protocol for the management of metabolic toxicities.

Table 1 Common Toxicity Criteria (CTC)

Adverse Event	Grade 0	Grade 1
Allergy/Immunology		
Allergic reaction/ hypersensitivity (including drug fever)	none	transient rash, drug fever < 38°C (< 100.4°F)
Note: Isolated urticaria, in the absence of other manifestations of an allergic or hypersensitivity reaction, is graded in the DERMATOLOGY/SKIN category.		
Allergic rhinitis (including sneezing, nasal stuffiness, postnasal drip)	none	mild, not requiring treatment
Autoimmune reaction	none	serologic or other evidence of autoimmune reaction but patient is asymptomatic (e.g., vitiligo), all organ function is normal and no treatment is required
Also consider Hypothyroidism, Colitis, Hemoglobin, Hemolysis.		
Serum sickness	none	—
Urticaria is graded in the DERMATOLOGY/SKIN category if it occurs as an isolated symptom. If it occurs with other manifestations of allergic or hypersensitivity reaction, grade as Allergic reaction/hypersensitivity above.		
Vasculitis	none	mild, not requiring treatment
Allergy/Immunology - Other (Specify, _____)	none	mild

	Grade	
2	**3**	**4**
Allergy/Immunology		
urticaria, drug fever ≥ 38°C (≥ 100.4°F), and/or asymptomatic bronchospasm	symptomatic bronchospasm, requiring parenteral medication(s), with or without urticaria; allergy-related edema/angioedema	anaphylaxis
moderate, requiring treatment	—	—
evidence of autoimmune reaction involving a nonessential organ or function (e.g., hypothyroidism), requiring treatment other than immunosuppressive drugs	reversible autoimmune reaction involving function of a major organ or other adverse event (e.g., transient colitis or anemia), requiring short-term immunosuppressive treatment	autoimmune reaction causing major grade 4 organ dysfunction; progressive and irreversible reaction; long-term administration of high-dose immunosuppressive therapy required
—	present	—
symptomatic, requiring medication	requiring steroids	ischemic changes or requiring amputation
moderate	severe	life-threatening or disabling

Table 1 Common Toxicity Criteria (CTC) *Continued*

Adverse Event	Grade 0	Grade 1
Auditory/Hearing		
Conductive hearing loss is graded as Middle ear/hearing in the AUDITORY/HEARING category.		
Earache is graded in the PAIN category.		
External auditory canal	normal	external otitis with erythema or dry desquamation
Note: Changes associated with radiation to external ear (pinnae) are graded under Radiation dermatitis in the DERMATOLOGY/SKIN category.		
Inner ear/hearing	normal	hearing loss on audiometry only
Middle ear/hearing	normal	serous otitis without subjective decrease in hearing
Auditory/Hearing - Other (Specify, _____)	normal	mild
Blood/Bone Marrow		
Bone marrow cellularity	normal for age	mildly hypocellular or ≤ 25% reduction from normal cellularity for age
Normal ranges: *children (≤ 18 years)*	*90% cellularity average*	
younger adults (19–59)	60–70% cellularity average	
older adults (≥ 60 years)	50% cellularity average	

	Grade	
2	**3**	**4**
Auditory/Hearing		
external otitis with moist desquamation	external otitis with discharge, mastoiditis	necrosis of the canal soft tissue or bone
tinnitus or hearing loss, not requiring hearing aid or treatment	tinnitus or hearing loss, correctable with hearing aid or treatment	severe unilateral or bilateral hearing loss (deafness), not correctable
serous otitis or infection requiring medical intervention; subjective decrease in hearing; rupture of tympanic membrane with discharge	otitis with discharge, mastoiditis or conductive hearing loss	necrosis of the canal soft tissue or bone
moderate	severe	life-threatening or disabling
Blood/Bone Marrow		
moderately hypocellular or > 25–≤ 50% reduction from normal cellularity for age or > 2 but < 4 weeks to recovery of normal bone marrow cellularity	severely hypocellular or > 50–≤ 75% reduction in cellularity for age or 4–6 weeks to recovery of normal bone marrow cellularity	aplasia or > 6 weeks to recovery of normal bone marrow cellularity

Table 1 Common Toxicity Criteria (CTC) *Continued*

		Grade
Adverse Event	**0**	**1**
Blood/Bone Marrow		
CD4 count	WNL	$<$LLN – 500/mm^3
Haptoglobin	normal	decreased
Hemoglobin (Hgb)	WNL	$<$LLN – 10.0 g/dL $<$LLN – 100 g/L $<$LLN – 6.2 mmol/L
For leukemia studies or bone marrow infiltrative/ myelophthisic processes, if specified in the protocol.	WNL	10 – $<$ 25% decrease from pretreatment
Hemolysis (e.g., immune hemolytic anemia, drug-related hemolysis, other)	none	only laboratory evidence of hemolysis [e.g., direct antiglobulin test (DAT, Coombs') schistocytes]
Leukocytes (total WBC)	WNL	$<$LLN – 3.0 × 10^9/L $<$LLN – 3000/mm^3
For BMT studies, if specified in the protocol.	WNL	$\geq$ 2.0 – $<$ 3.0 × 10^9/L $\geq$ 2000 – $<$ 3000/mm^3
For pediatric BMT studies (using age, race, and sex normal values), if specified in the protocol.		$\geq$ 75 – $<$ 100% LLN
Lymphopenia	WNL	$<$LLN – 1.0 × 10^9/L $<$LLN – 1000/mm^3
For pediatric BMT studies (using age, race, and sex normal values), if specified in the protocol.		$\geq$ 75 – $<$ 100% LLN

	Grade	
2	**3**	**4**
	Blood/Bone Marrow	
200–< 500/mm^3	50 – < 200/mm^3	< 50/mm^3
—	absent	—
8.0 – < 10.0 g/dL	65 – < 8.0 g/dL	< 6.5 g/dL
8.0 – < 100 g/L	65 – < 80 g/L	< 65 g/L
4.9 – < 6.2 mmol/L	4.0 – < 4.9 mmol/L	< 4.0 mmol/L
25 – < 50% decrease from pretreatment	50 – < 75% decrease from pretreatment	≥ 75% decrease from pretreatment
evidence of red cell destruction and ≥ 2 gm decrease in hemoglobin, no transfusion	requiring transfusion and/or medical intervention (e.g., steroids)	catastrophic consequences of hemolysis (e.g., renal failure, hypotension, bronchospasm, emergency splenectomy)
≥ 2.0 – < 3.0 × 10^9/L	≥ 1.0 – < 2.0 × 10^9/L	< 1.0 × 10^9/L
≥ 2000 – < 3000/mm^3	≥ 1000 – < 2000/mm^3	< 1000/mm^3
≥ 1.0 – < 2.0 × 10^9/L	≥ 0.5 – < 1.0 × 10^9/L	< 0.5 × 10^9/L
≥ 1000 – < 2000/mm^3	≥ 500 – < 1000/mm^3	< 500/mm^3
≥ 50 – < 75% LLN	≥ 25 – < 50% LLN	< 25% LLN
≥ 0.5 – < 1.0 × 10^9/L	< 0.5 × 10^9/L	—
≥ 500 – < 1000/mm^3	< 500/mm^3	
≥ 50 – < 75% LLN	≥ 25 – < 75% LLN	< 25% LLN

Table 1 Common Toxicity Criteria (CTC) *Continued*

Adverse Event	Grade 0	Grade 1
Blood/Bone Marrow		
Neutrophils/granulocytes (ANC/AGC)	WNL	$\geq 1.5 - < 2.0 \times 10^9/L$ $\geq 1500 - < 2000/mm^3$
For BMT studies, if specified in the protocol.	WNL	$\geq 1.0 - < 1.5 \times 10^9/L$ $\geq 1000 - < 1500/mm^3$
For leukemia studies or bone marrow infiltrative/ myelophthisic process, if specified in the protocol.	WNL	10 – < 25% decrease from baseline
Platelets	WNL	$< LLN - 75.0 \times 10^9/L$ $< LLN - 75,000/mm^3$
For BMT studies, if specified in the protocol.	WNL	$\geq 50.0 - < 75.0 \times 10^9/L$ $\geq 50,000 - < 75,000 \ mm^3$
For leukemia studies or bone marrow infiltrative/ myelophthisic process, if specified in the protocol.	WNL	10 – < 25% decrease from baseline
Transfusion: Platelets	none	—
For BMT studies, if specified in the protocol.	none	1 platelet transfusion in 24 hours

	Grade	
2	**3**	**4**
Blood/Bone Marrow		
$\geq 1.0 - < 1.5 \times 10^9/L$	$\geq 0.5 - < 1.0 \times 10^9/L$	$< 0.5 \times 10^9/L$
$\geq 1000 - < 1500/mm^3$	$\geq 500 - < 1000/mm^3$	$< 500/mm^3$
$\geq 0.5 - < 1.0 \times 10^9/L$	$\geq 0.1 - < 0.5 \times 10^9/L$	$< 0.1 \times 10^9/L$
$\geq 500 - < 1000/mm^3$	$\geq 100 - < 500/mm^3$	$< 100/mm^3$
25 – < 50% decrease from baseline	50 – < 75% decrease from baseline	$\geq 75\%$ decrease from baseline
$\geq 50.0 - < 75.0 \times 10^9/L$	$\geq 10.0 - < 50.0 \times 10^9/L$	$< 10.0 \times 10^9/L$
$\geq 50,000 - < 75,000/mm^3$	$\geq 10,000 - < 50,000/mm^3$	$< 10,000/mm^3$
$\geq 20.0 - < 50.0 \times 10^9/L$	$\geq 10.0 - < 20.0 \times 10^9/L$	$< 10.0 \times 10^9/L$
$\geq 20,000 - < 50,000/mm^3$	$\geq 10,000 - < 20,000/mm^3$	$< 10,000/mm^3$
25 – < 50% decrease from baseline	50 – < 75% decrease from baseline	$\geq 75\%$ decrease from baseline
—	yes	platelet transfusions and other measures required to improve platelet increment; platelet transfusion refractoriness associated with life-threatening bleeding (e.g., HLA or cross matched platelet transfusions)
2 platelet transfusions in 24 hours	≥ 3 platelet transfusions in 24 hours	platelet transfusions and other measures required to improve platelet increment; platelet transfusion refractoriness associated with life-threatening bleeding (e.g., HLA or cross matched platelet transfusions)

Table 1 Common Toxicity Criteria (CTC) *Continued*

Adverse Event	Grade 0	Grade 1
Blood/Bone Marrow		
Transfusion: pRBCs	none	—
For BMT studies, if specified in the protocol.	none	≤ 2 u pRBC in 24 hours elective or planned
For pediatric BMT studies, if specified in the protocol.	*none*	*≤ 15mL/kg in 24 hours elective or planned*
Blood/Bone Marrow - Other (Specify, _____)	none	mild
Cardiovascular (Arrhythmia)		
Conduction abnormality/ Atrioventricular heart block	none	asymptomatic, not requiring treatment (e.g., Mobitz type I second-degree AV block, Wenckebach)
Nodal/junctional arrhythmia/dysrhythmia	none	asymptomatic, not requiring treatment
Palpitations	none	present
Note: Grade palpitations *only* in the absence of a documented arrhythmia.		
Prolonged QTc interval (QTc > 0.48 seconds)	none	asymptomatic, not requiring treatment
Sinus bradycardia	none	asymptomatic, not requiring treatment

	Grade	
2	**3**	**4**
Blood/Bone Marrow		
—	yes	—
3 u pRBC in 24 hours elective or planned	≥ 4 u pRBC in 24 hours	hemorrhage or hemolysis associated with life-threatening anemia; medical intervention required to improve hemoglobin
> 15 – ≤ 30mL/kg in 24 hours elective or planned	*> 30mL/kg in 24 hours*	*hemorrhage or hemolysis associated with life-threatening anemia; medical intervention required to improve hemoglobin*
moderate	severe	life-threatening or disabling
Cardiovascular (Arrhythmia)		
symptomatic, but not requiring treatment	symptomatic and requiring treatment (e.g., Mobitz type II second-degree AV block, third-degree AV block)	life-threatening (e.g., arrhythmia associated with CHF, hypotension, syncope, shock)
symptomatic, but not requiring treatment	symptomatic and requiring treatment	life-threatening (e.g., arrhythmia associated with CHF, hypotension, syncope, shock)
—	—	—
symptomatic, but not requiring treatment	symptomatic and requiring treatment	life-threatening (e.g., arrhythmia associated with CHF, hypotension, syncope, shock)
symptomatic, but not requiring treatment	symptomatic and requiring treatment	life-threatening (e.g., arrhythmia associated with CHF, hypotension, syncope, shock)

Table 1 Common Toxicity Criteria (CTC) *Continued*

| | Grade | |
Adverse Event	0	1
Cardiovascular (Arrhythmia)		
Sinus tachycardia	none	asymptomatic, not requiring treatment
Supraventricular arrhythmias (SVT/ atrial fibrillation/flutter)	none	asymptomatic, not requiring treatment
Syncope (fainting) is graded in the NEUROLOGY category.		
Vasovagal episode	none	—
Ventricular arrhythmia (PVCs/bigeminy/ trigeminy/ventricular tachycardia)	none	asymptomatic, not requiring treatment
Cardiovascular/ Arrhythmia - Other (Specify, _____)	none	asymptomatic, not requiring treatment
Cardiovascular (General)		
Acute vascular leak syndrome	absent	—
Cardiac-ischemia/ infarction	none	non-specific T-wave flattening or changes
Cardiac left ventricular function	normal	asymptomatic decline of resting ejection fraction of $\geq 10\%$ but $< 20\%$ of baseline value; shortening fraction $\geq 24\%$ but $< 30\%$

	Grade	
2	**3**	**4**
Cardiovascular (Arrhythmia)		
symptomatic, but not requiring treatment	symptomatic and requiring treatment of underlying cause	—
symptomatic, but not requiring treatment	symptomatic and requiring treatment	life-threatening (e.g., arrhythmia associated with CHF, hypotension, syncope, shock)
present without loss of consciousness	present with loss of consciousness	—
symptomatic, but not requiring treatment	symptomatic and requiring treatment	life-threatening (e.g., arrhythmia associated with CHF, hypotension, syncope, shock)
symptomatic, but not requiring treatment	symptomatic and requiring treatment of underlying cause	life-threatening (e.g., arrhythmia associated with CHF, hypotension, syncope, shock)
Cardiovascular (General)		
symptomatic, but not requiring fluid support	respiratory compromise or requiring fluids	life-threatening; requiring pressor support and/or ventilatory support
asymptomatic, ST- and T-wave changes suggesting ischemia	angina without evidence of infarction	acute myocardial infarction
asymptomatic but resting ejection fraction below LLN for laboratory or decline of resting ejection fraction ≥ 20% of baseline value; < 24% shortening fraction	CHF responsive to treatment	severe or refractory CHF or requiring intubation

Table 1 Common Toxicity Criteria (CTC) *Continued*

Adverse Event	0	Grade 1
Cardiovascular (General)		
CNS cerebrovascular ischemia is graded in the NEUROLOGY category.		
Cardiac troponin I (cTnI)	normal	—
Cardiac troponin T (cTnT)	normal	≥ 0.03 – < 0.05 ng/mL
Edema	none	asymptomatic, not requiring therapy
Hypertension	none	asymptomatic, transient increase by > 20 mmHg (diastolic) or to > 150/100 * if previously WNL; not requiring treatment
*Note: For pediatric patients, use age and sex appropriate normal values. >95th percentile ULN.		
Hypotension	none	changes, but not requiring therapy (including transient orthostatic hypotension)

Also consider Syncope (fainting)

Notes: Angina or MI is graded as Cardiac-ischemia/infarction in the
       CARDIOVASCULAR (GENERAL) category.

*For pediatric patients, systolic BP 65 mmHg or less in infants up to 1 year old and
70 mmHg or less in children older than 1 year of age, use two successive or three
measurements in 24 hours.*

Myocarditis	none	—

	Grade	
2	**3**	**4**
Cardiovascular (General)		
—	levels consistent with unstable angina as defined by the manufacturer	levels consistent with myocardial infarction as defined by the manufacturer
$\geq 0.05 - < 0.1$ ng/mL	$\geq 0.1 - < 0.2$ ng/mL	≥ 0.2 ng/mL
symptomatic, requiring therapy	symptomatic edema limiting function and unresponsive to therapy or requiring drug discontinuation	anasarca (severe generalized edema)
recurrent or persistent or symptomatic increase by > 20 mmHg (diastolic) or to $> 150/100$ * if previously WNL; not requiring treatment	requiring therapy or more intensive therapy than previously	hypertensive crisis
requiring brief fluid replacement or other therapy but not hospitalization; no physiologic consequences	requiring therapy and sustained medical attention, but resolves without persisting physiologic consequences	shock (associated with acidermia and impairing vital organ function due to tissue hypoperfusion)
—	CHF responsive to treatment	severe or refractory CHF

Table 1 Common Toxicity Criteria (CTC) *Continued*

Adverse Event	Grade 0	Grade 1
Cardiovascular (General)		
Operative injury of vein/artery	none	primary suture repair for injury, but not requiring transfusion
Pericardial effusion/ pericarditis	none	asymptomatic effusion, not requiring treatment
Peripheral arterial ischemia	none	—
Phlebitis (superficial)	none	—
Notes: Injection site reaction is graded in the DERMATOLOGY/SKIN category.		
Thrombosis/embolism is graded in the CARDIOVASCULAR (GENERAL) category.		
Syncope (fainting) is graded in the NEUROLOGY category.		
Thrombosis/embolism	none	—
Vein/artery operative injury is graded as Operative injury of vein/artery in the CARDIOVASCULAR (GENERAL) category.		
Visceral arterial ischemia (non-myocardial)	none	—
Cardiovascular/General - Other (Specify, _____)	none	mild

	Grade	
2	**3**	**4**
Cardiovascular (General)		
primary suture repair for injury, requiring transfusion	vascular occlusion requiring surgery or bypass for injury	myocardial infarction; resection of organ (e.g., bowel, limb)
pericarditis (rub, ECG changes, and/or chest pain)	with physiologic consequences	tamponade (drainage or pericardial window required)
brief episode of ischemia managed nonsurgically and without permanent deficit	requiring surgical intervention	life-threatening or with permanent functional deficit (e.g., amputation)
present	—	—
deep vein thrombosis, not requiring anticoagulant	deep vein thrombosis, requiring anticoagulant therapy	embolic event including pulmonary embolism
brief episode of ischemia managed nonsurgically and without permanent deficit	requiring surgical intervention	life-threatening or with permanent functional deficit (e.g., resection of ileum)
moderate	severe	life-threatening or disabling

Table 1 Common Toxicity Criteria (CTC) *Continued*

Adverse Event	Grade 0	Grade 1
Coagulation		
Note: See the HEMORRHAGE category for grading the severity of bleeding events.		
DIC (dissseminated intravascular coagulation)	absent	—
Note: Must have increased fibrin split products or D-dimer in order to grade as DIC.		
Fibrinogen	WNL	$\geq 0.75 - < 1.0 \times$ LLN
For leukemia studies or bone marrow infiltrative/myelophthisic process, if specified in the protocol.	WNL	< 20% decrease from pretreatment value or LLN
Partial thromboplastin time (PTT)	WNL	$> $ ULN $- \leq 1.5 \times$ ULN
Phlebitis is graded in the CARDIOVASCULAR (GENERAL) category.		
Prothrombin time (PT)	WNL	$> $ ULN $- \leq 1.5 \times$ ULN
Thrombosis/embolism is graded in the CARDIOVASCULAR (GENERAL) category.		
Thrombotic microangiopathy (e.g., thrombotic thrombocytopenic purpura/TTP or hemolytic uremic syndrome/HUS)	absent	—
For BMT studies, if specified in the protocol.		evidence of RBC destruction (schistocytosis) without clinical consequences
Note: Must have microangiopathic changes on blood smear (e.g., schistocytes, helmet cells, red cell fragments).		
Coagulation – Other (Specify, _____)	none	mild

	Grade	
2	**3**	**4**
	Coagulation	
—	laboratory findings present with *no* bleeding	laboratory finding *and* bleeding
$\geq 0.5 - < 0.75 \times$ LLN	$\geq 0.25 - < 0.5 \times$ LLN	$< 0.25 \times$ LLN
$\geq 20 - < 40\%$ decrease from pretreatment value or LLN	$\geq 40 - < 70\%$ decrease from pretreatment value or LLN	< 50 mg
$> 1.5 - \leq 2 \times$ ULN	$> 2 \times$ ULN	—
$> 1.5 - \leq 2 \times$ ULN	$> 2 \times$ ULN	—
—	laboratory findings present without clinical consequences	laboratory findings and clinical consequences, (e.g., CNS hemorrhage/ bleeding or thrombosis/ embolism or renal failure) requiring therapeutic intervention
evidence of RBC destruction with elevated creatinine ($\leq 3 \times$ ULN)	evidence of RBC destruction with creatinine ($> 3 \times$ ULN) not requiring dialysis	evidence of RBC destruction with renal failure requiring dialysis and/or encephalopathy
moderate	severe	life-threatening or disabling

Table 1 Common Toxicity Criteria (CTC) *Continued*

Adverse Event	Grade 0	Grade 1
Constitutional Symptoms		
Fatigue (lethargy, malaise, asthenia)	none	increased fatigue over baseline, but not altering normal activities
Fever (in the absence of neutropenia, where neutropenia is defined as AGC $< 1.0 \times 10^9$/L)	none	38.0 – 39.0°C (100.4 – 102.2°F)
Also consider Allergic reaction/hypersensitivity.		
Note: The temperature measurements listed above are oral or tympanic.		
Hot flashes/flushes are graded in the ENDOCRINE category.		
Rigors, chills	none	mild, requiring symptomatic treatment (e.g., blanket) or non-narcotic medication
Sweating (diaphoresis)	normal	mild and occasional
Weight gain	< 5%	5 – < 10%
Also consider Ascites, Edema, Pleural effusion (non-malignant).		
Weight gain associated with Veno-occlusive Disease (VOD) for BMT studies, if specified in the protocol.	< 2%	$\geq 2 - < 5\%$
Also consider Ascites, Edema, Pleural effusion (non-malignant).		
Weight loss	< 5%	5 – < 10%
Also consider Vomiting, Dehydration, Diarrhea.		
Constitutional Symptoms - Other (Specify, _____)	none	mild

	Grade	
2	**3**	**4**
Constitutional Symptoms		
moderate (e.g., decrease in performance status by 1 ECOG level *or* 20% Karnofsky or Lansky) *or* causing difficulty performing some activities	severe (e.g., decrease in performance status by ≥ 2 ECOG levels *or* 40% Karnofsky or Lansky) *or* loss of ability to perform some activities	bedridden or disabling
39.1 – 40.0°C (102.3 – 104.0°F)	> 40.0%C (> 104.0°F) for < 24 hrs	> 40.0°C (> 104.0°F) for > 24 hrs
severe and/or prolonged, requiring narcotic medication	not responsive to narcotic medication	—
frequent or drenching	—	—
10 – < 20%	≥ 20%	—
≥ 5 – < 10%	≥ 10% or as ascites	≥ 10% or fluid retention resulting in pulmonary failure
10 – < 20%	≥ 20%	—
moderate	severe	life-threatening or disabling

Table 1 Common Toxicity Criteria (CTC) *Continued*

Adverse Event	Grade 0	Grade 1
Dermatology/Skin		
Alopecia	normal	mild hair loss
Bruising (in absence of grade 3 or 4 thrombocytopenia)	none	localized or in dependent area
Note: Bruising *resulting from grade 3 or 4 thrombocytopenia* is graded as Petechiae/ purpura *and* Hemorrhage/bleeding with grade 3 or 4 thrombocytopenia in the HEMORRHAGE category, *not* in the DERMATOLOGY/SKIN category.		
Dry skin	normal	controlled with emollients
Erythema multiforme (e.g., Stevens-Johnson syndrome, toxic epidermal necrolysis)	absent	—
Flushing	absent	present
Hand-foot skin reaction	none	skin changes or dermatitis without pain (e.g., erythema, peeling)
Injection site reaction	none	pain or itching or erythema
Nail changes	normal	discoloration or ridging (koilonychia) or pitting
Petechiae is graded in the HEMORRHAGE category.		
Photosensitivity	none	painless erytherma
Pigmentation changes (e.g., vitiligo)	none	localized pigmentation changes

	Grade	
2	**3**	**4**
Dermatology/Skin		
pronounced hair loss	—	—
generalized	—	—
not controlled with emollients	—	—
scattered, but not generalized eruption	severe or requiring IV fluids (e.g., generalized rash or painful stomatitis)	life-threatening (e.g., exfoliative or ulcerating dermatitis or requiring enteral or parenteral nutritional support)
—	—	—
skin changes with pain, not interfering with function	skin changes with pain, interfering with function	—
pain or swelling, with inflammation or phlebitis	ulceration or necrosis that is severe or prolonged, or requiring surgery	—
partial or complete loss of nail(s) or pain in nailbeds	—	—
painful erytherma	erythema with desquamation	—
generalized pigmentation changes	—	—

Table 1 Common Toxicity Criteria (CTC) *Continued*

Adverse Event	Grade 0	Grade 1
Dermatology/Skin		
Pruritus	none	mild or localized, relieved spontaneously or by local measures
Purpura is graded in the HEMORRHAGE category.		
Radiation dermatitis	none	faint erythema or dry desquamation
Note: Pain associated with radiation dermatitis is graded separately in the PAIN category as Pain due to radiation.		
Radiation recall reaction (reaction following chemotherapy in the absence of additional radiation therapy that occurs in a previous radiation port)	none	faint erythema or dry desquamation
Rash/desquamation	none	macular or papular eruption or erythema without associated symptoms
Note: Stevens-Johnson syndrome is graded separately as Erythema multiforme in the DERMATOLOGY/SKIN category.		
Rash/dermatitis associated with high-dose chemotherapy or BMT studies.	none	faint erythema or dry desquamation

	Grade	
2	**3**	**4**
Dermatology/Skin		
intense or widespread, relieved spontaneously or by systemic measures	intense or widespread, and poorly controlled despite treatment	—
moderate to brisk erythema or a patchy moist desquamation, mostly confined to skin folds and creases; moderate edema	confluent moist desquamation ≥ 1.5 cm diameter and not confined to skin folds; pitting edema	skin necrosis or ulceration of full thickness dermis; may include bleeding not induced by minor trauma or abrasion
moderate to brisk erythema or a patchy moist desquamation, mostly confined to skin folds and creases; moderate edema	confluent moist desquamation ≥ 1.5 cm diameter and not confined to skin folds; pitting edema	skin necrosis or ulceration of full thickness dermis; may include bleeding not induced by minor trauma or abrasion
macular or papular eruption or erythema with pruritus or other associated symptoms covering < 50% of body surface or localized desquamation or other lesions covering < 50% of body surface area	symptomatic generalized erythroderma or macular, papular or vesicular eruption or desquamation covering ≥ 50% of body surface area	generalized exfoliative dermatitis or ulcerative dermatitis
moderate to brisk erythema or a patchy moist desquamation, mostly confined to skin folds and creases; moderate edema	confluent moist desquamation ≥ 1.5 cm diameter and not confined to skin folds; pitting edema	skin necrosis or ulceration of full thickness dermis; may include spontaneous bleeding not induced by minor trauma or abrasion

Table 1 Common Toxicity Criteria (CTC) *Continued*

Adverse Event	Grade 0	Grade 1
Dermatology/Skin		
Rash/desquamation associated with graft versus host disease (GVHD) for BMT studies, if specified in the protocol.	none	macular or papular eruption or erythema covering < 25% of body surface area without associated symptoms
Note: Stevens-Johnson syndrome is graded separately as Erythema multiforme in the DERMATOLOGY/SKIN category.		
Urticaria (hives, welts, wheals)	none	requiring no medication
Wound-infectious	none	cellulitis
Wound-non-infectious	none	incisional separation
Dermatology/Skin - Other (Specify, _____)	none	mild
Endocrine		
Cushingoid appearance (e.g., moon face, buffalo hump, centripetal obesity, cutaneous striae)	absent	—
Feminization of male	absent	—
Gynecomastia	none	mild
Hot flashes/flushes	none	mild or no more than 1 per day

	Grade	
2	3	4
Dermatology/Skin		
macular or papular eruption or erythema with pruritus or other associated symptoms covering ≥ 25% – < 50% of body surface or localized desquamation or other lesions covering ≥ 25 – < 50% of body surface area	symptomatic generalized erythroderma or symptomatic macular, papular or vesicular eruption, with bullous formation, or desquamation covering ≥ 50% of body surface area	generalized exfoliative dermatitis or ulcerative dermatitis or bullous formation
requiring PO or topical treatment or IV medication or steroids for < 24 hours	requiring IV medication or steroids for ≥ 24 hours	—
superficial infection	infection requiring IV antibiotics	necrotizing fasciitis
incisional hernia	fascial disruption without evisceration	fascial disruption with evisceration
moderate	severe	life-threatening or disabling
Endocrine		
present	—	—
—	present	—
pronounced or painful	pronounced or painful and requiring surgery	—
moderate and greater than 1 per day	—	—

Table 1 Common Toxicity Criteria (CTC) *Continued*

Adverse Event	Grade 0	Grade 1
Endocrine		
Hypothyroidism	absent	asymptomatic, TSH elevated, no therapy given
Masculinization of female	absent	—
SIADH (syndrome of inappropriate antidiuretic hormone)	absent	—
Endocrine—Other (Specify, _____)	none	mild
Gastrointestinal		
Amylase is graded in the METABOLIC/LABORATORY category.		
Anorexia	none	loss of appetite
Ascites (non-malignant)	none	asymptomatic
Colitis	none	—
Constipation	none	requiring stool softener or dietary modification
Dehydration	none	dry mucous membranes and/or dimished skin turgor

	Grade	
2	3	4
Endocrine		
symptomatic or thyroid replacement treatment given	patient hospitalized for manifestation of hypothyroidism	myxedema coma
—	present	—
—	present	—
moderate	severe	life-threatening or disabling
Gastrointestinal		
oral intake significantly decreased	requiring IV fluids	requiring feeding tube or parenteral nutrition
symptomatic, requiring diuretics	symptomatic, requiring therapeutic paracentesis	life-threatening physiologic consequences
abdominal pain with mucus and/or blood in stool	abdominal pain, fever, change in bowel habits with ileus or peritoneal signs, and radiographic or biopsy documentation	perforation or requiring surgery or toxic megacolon
requiring laxatives	obstipation requiring manual evacuation or enema	obstruction or toxic megacolon
requiring IV fluid replacement (brief)	requiring IV fluid replacement (sustained)	physiologic consequences requiring intensive care; hemodynamic collapse

Table 1 Common Toxicity Criteria (CTC) *Continued*

		Grade
Adverse Event	**0**	**1**
Gastrointestinal		
Diarrhea patients without colostomy:	none	increase of < 4 stools/day over pretreatment
patients with a colostomy:	none	mild increase in loose, watery colostomy output compared with pretreatment
Diarrhea associated with graft versus host disease (GVHD) for BMT studies, if specified in the protocol.	none	> 500 – ≤ 1000mL of diarrhea/day
For pediatric BMT studies, if specified in the protocol.		*> 5 – ≤ 10 mL/kg of diarrhea/day*
Duodenal ulcer (requires radiographic or endoscopic documentation)	none	—
Dyspepsia/heartburn	none	mild
Dysphagia, esophagitis, odynophagia (painful swallowing)	none	mild dysphagia, but can eat regular diet

Note: If the adverse event is radiation-related, grade *either* under Dysphagia-esophageal related to radiation *or* Dysphagia-pharyngeal related to radiation.

	Grade	
2	**3**	**4**
Gastrointestinal		
increase of 4–6 stools/day, or nocturnal stools	increase of ≥ 7 stools/ day or incontinence; or need for parenteral support for dehydration	physiologic consequences requiring intensive care; or hemodynamic collapse
moderate increase in loose, water colostomy output compared with pretreatment, but not interfering with normal activity	severe increase in loose, watery colostomy output compared with pretreatment, interfering with normal activity	physiologic consequences requiring intensive care; or hemodynamic collapse
> 1000 – ≤ 1500mL of diarrhea/day	> 1500mL of diarrhea/day	severe abdominal pain with or without ileus
> 10 – ≤ 15 mL/kg of diarrhea/day	*> 15 mL/kg of diarrhea/day*	—
requiring medical management or nonsurgical treatment	uncontrolled by outpatient medical management; requiring hospitalization	perforation or bleeding, requiring emergency surgery
moderate	severe	—
dysphagia, requiring predominantly pureed, soft, or liquid diet	dysphagia, requiring IV hydration	complete obstruction (cannot swallow saliva) requiring enteral or parenteral nutritional support, or perforation

Table 1 Common Toxicity Criteria (CTC) *Continued*

		Grade
Adverse Event	**0**	**1**
	Gastrointestinal	
Dysphagia-*esophageal* related to radiation	none	mild dysphagia, but can eat regular diet
Note: Fistula is graded separately as Fistula-esophageal.		
Dysphagia-*pharyngeal* related to radiation	none	mild dysphagia, but can eat regular diet
Note: Fistula is graded separately as Fistula-pharyngeal.		
Fistula-esophageal	none	—
Fistula-intestinal	none	—
Fistula-pharyngeal	none	—
Fistula-rectal/anal	none	—
Flatulence	none	mild
Gastric ulcer (requires radiographic or endoscopic documentation)	none	—

	Grade	
2	**3**	**4**
Gastrointestinal		
dysphagia, requiring predominantly pureed, soft, or liquid diet	dysphagia, requiring feeding tube, IV hydration or hyperalimentation	complete obstruction (cannot swallow saliva); ulceration with bleeding not induced by minor trauma or abrasion or perforation
dysphagia, requiring predominantly pureed, soft, or liquid diet	dysphagia, requiring feeding tube, IV hydration or hyperalimentation	complete obstruction (cannot swallow saliva); ulceration with bleeding not induced by minor trauma or abrasion or perforation
—	present	requiring surgery
—	present	requiring surgery
—	present	requiring surgery
—	present	requiring surgery
moderate	—	—
requiring medical management or nonsurgical treatment	bleeding without perforation, uncontrolled by outpatient medical management; requiring hospitalization or surgery	perforation or bleeding, requiring emergency surgery

Table 1 Common Toxicity Criteria (CTC) *Continued*

		Grade
Adverse Event	**0**	**1**
Gastrointestinal		
Gastritis	none	—
Hematemesis is graded in the HEMORRHAGE category.		
Hematochezia is graded in the HEMORRHAGE category as Rectal bleeding/hematochezia.		
Ileus (or neuroconstipation)	none	—
Mouth dryness	normal	mild

Mucositis

Notes: Mucositis *not due to radiation* is graded in the GASTROINTESTINAL category
  for specific sites: Colitis, Esophagitis, Gastritis, Stomatitis/pharyngitis
  (oral/pharyngeal mucositis), and Typhlitis; or the RENAL/GENITOURINARY
  category for Vaginitis.

  Radiation-related mucositis is graded as Mucositis due to radiation.

Mucositis due to radiation	none	erythema of the mucosa

Note: Grade radiation mucositis of the larynx here.

  Dysphagia related to radiation is also graded as *either* Dysphagia-esophageal
  related to radiation *or* Dysphagia-pharyngeal related to radiation,
  depending on the site of treatment.

Nausea	none	able to eat

| | Grade | |
2	3	4
Gastrointestinal		
requiring medical management or nonsurgical treatment	uncontrolled by outpatient medical management; requiring hospitalization or surgery	life-threatening bleeding, requiring emergency surgery
intermittent, not requiring intervention	requiring non-surgical intervention	requiring surgery
moderate	—	—
patchy pseudomembranous reaction (patches generally ≤ 1.5 cm in diameter and noncontiguous)	confluent pseudomembranous reaction (contiguous patches generally > 1.5 cm in diameter)	necrosis or deep ulceration; may include bleeding not induced by minor trauma or abrasion
oral intake significantly decreased	no significant intake, requiring IV fluids	—

Table 1 Common Toxicity Criteria (CTC) *Continued*

| | | Grade |
Adverse Event	0	1
Gastrointestinal		
Pancreatitis	none	—
Note: Amylase is graded in the METABOLIC/LABORATORY category.		
Pharyngitis is graded in the GASTROINTESTINAL category as Stomatitis/ pharyngitis (oral/pharyngeal mucositis).		
Proctitis	none	increased stool frequency, occasional blood-streaked stools or rectal discomfort (including hemorrhoids) not requiring medication
Notes: Fistula is graded separately as Fistula-rectal/anal.		
Salivary gland changes	none	slightly thickened saliva; may have slightly altered taste (e.g., metallic); additional fluids may be required
Sense of smell	normal	slightly altered
Stomatitis/pharyngitis (oral/pharyngeal mucositis)	none	painless ulcers, erythema, or mild soreness in the absence of lesions
For BMT studies, if specified in the protocol.	none	painless ulcers, erythema, or mild soreness in the absence of lesions
Note: Radiation-related mucositis is graded as Mucositis due to radiation.		

	Grade	
2	**3**	**4**
Gastrointestinal		
—	abdominal pain with pancreatic enzyme elevation	complicated by shock (acute circulatory failure)
increased stool frequency, bleeding, mucus discharge, or rectal discomfort requiring medication; anal fissure	increased stool frequency/diarrhea requiring parenteral support; rectal bleeding requiring transfusion; or persistent mucus discharge, necessitating pads	perforation, bleeding or necrosis or other life-threatening complication requiring surgical intervention (e.g., colostomy)
thick, ropy, sticky saliva; markedly altered taste; alteration in diet required	—	acute salivary gland necrosis
markedly altered	—	—
painful erythema, edema, or ulcers but can eat or swallow	painful erythema, edema, or ulcers requiring IV hydration	severe ulceration or requires parenteral or enteral nutritional support or prophylactic intubation
painful erythema, edema or ulcers but can swallow	painful erythema, edema, or ulcers preventing swallowing or requiring hydration or parenteral (or enteral) nutritional support	severe ulceration requiring prophylactic intubation or resulting in documented aspiration pneumonia

Table 1 Common Toxicity Criteria (CTC) *Continued*

		Grade
Adverse Event	**0**	**1**
Gastrointestinal		
Taste disturbance (dysgeusia)	normal	slightly altered
Typhlitis (inflammation of the cecum)	none	—
Vomiting	none	1 episode in 24 hours over pretreatment
Weight gain is graded in the CONSTITUTIONAL SYMPTOMS category.		
Weight loss is graded in the CONSTITUTIONAL SYMPTOMS category.		
Gastrointestinal—Other (Specify, _____)	none	mild
Hemorrhage		

Notes: Transfusion in this section refers to pRBC infusion.

For *any* bleeding with grade 3 or 4 platelets (< 50,000), *always* grade Hemorrhage/ bleeding with grade 3 or 4 thrombocytopenia. Also consider Platelets, Transfusion: pRBCs, and Transfusion: platelets in addition to grading severity by grading the site or type of bleeding.

If the site or type of Hemorrhage/bleeding is listed, also use the grading that incorporates the site of bleeding: CNS Hemorrhage/bleeding, Hematuria, Hematemesis, Hemoptysis, Hemorrhage/bleeding with surgery, Melena/ lower GI bleeding, Petechiae/purpura (Hemorrhage/bleeding into skin), Rectal bleeding/hematochezia, Vaginal bleeding.

If the platelet count is ≥ 50,000 and the site or type of bleeding is listed, grade the specific site. If the site or type is *not* listed and the platelet count is ≥ 50,000, grade Hemorrhage/bleeding without grade 3 or 4 thrombo- cytopenia and specify the site or type in the OTHER category.

	Grade	
2	**3**	**4**
Gastrointestinal		
markedly altered	—	—
—	abdominal pain, diarrhea, fever, and radiographic or biopsy documentation	perforation, bleeding or necrosis or other life-threatening complication requiring surgical intervention (e.g., colostomy)
2–5 episodes in 24 hours over pretreatment	≥ 6 episodes in 24 hours over pretreatment; or need for IV fluids	requiring parenteral nutrition; or physiologic consequences requiring intensive care; hemodynamic collapse
moderate	severe	life-threatening or disabling
Hemorrhage		

Table 1 Common Toxicity Criteria (CTC) *Continued*

Adverse Event	Grade 0	Grade 1
Hemorrhage		
Hemorrhage/bleeding with grade 3 or 4 thrombocytopenia	none	mild without transfusion
Hemorrhage/bleeding without grade 3 or 4 thrombocytopenia	none	mild without transfusion
Note: Bleeding in the absence of grade 3 or 4 thrombocytopenia is graded here only if the specific site or type of bleeding is not listed elsewhere in the HEMORRHAGE category.		
CNS hemorrhage/ bleeding	none	—
Epistaxis	none	mild without transfusion
Hematemesis	none	mild without transfusion
Hematuria (in the absence of vaginal bleeding)	none	microscopic only
Hemoptysis	none	mild without transfusion

	Grade	
2	3	4
	Hemorrhage	
	requiring transfusion	catastrophic bleeding requiring major non-elective intervention
	requiring transfusion	catastrophic bleeding requiring major non-elective intervention
—	bleeding noted on CT or other scan with no clinical conseqences	hemorrhagic stroke or hemorrhagic vascular event (CVA) with neurologic signs and symptoms
—	requiring transfusion	catastrophic bleeding, requiring major non-elective intervention
—	requiring transfusion	catastrophic bleeding, requiring major non-elective intervention
intermittent gross bleeding, no clots	persistent gross bleeding or clots; may require catheterization or instrumentation, or transfusion	open surgery or necrosis or deep bladder ulceration
—	requiring transfusion	catastrophic bleeding, requiring major non-elective intervention

Table 1 Common Toxicity Criteria (CTC) *Continued*

		Grade
Adverse Event	**0**	**1**
Hemorrhage		
Hemorrhage/bleeding associated with surgery	none	mild without transfusion
Note: Expected blood loss at the time of surgery is not graded as an adverse event		
Melena/GI bleeding	none	mild without transfusion
Petechiae/purpura (hemorrhage/bleeding into skin or mucosa)	none	rare petechiae of skin
Rectal bleeding/ hematochezia	none	mild without transfusion or medication
Vaginal bleeding	none	spotting, requiring < 2 pads per day
Hemorrhage—Other (Specify site, _____)	none	mild without transfusion
Hepatic		
Alkaline phosphatase	WNL	> ULN – 2.5 × ULN
Bilirubin	WNL	> ULN – 1.5 × ULN
Bilirubin associated with graft versus host disease (GVHD) for BMT studies, if specified in the protocol.	normal	≥ 2 – < 3 mg/100 mL
GGT (γ - Glutamyl transpeptidase)	WNL	> ULN – 2.5 × ULN

	Grade	
2	**3**	**4**
Hemorrhage		
—	requiring transfusion	catastrophic bleeding, requiring major non-elective intervention
—	requiring transfusion	catastrophic bleeding, requiring major non-elective intervention
petechiae or purpura in dependent areas of skin	generalized petechiae or purpura of skin or petechiae of any musosal site	—
persistent, requiring medication (e.g., steroid suppositories) and/or break from radiation treatment	requiring transfusion	catastrophic bleeding, requiring major non-elective intervention
requiring ≥ 2 pads per day, but not requiring transfusion	requiring transfusion	catastrophic bleeding, requiring major non-elective intervention
—	requiring transfusion	catastrophic bleeding, requiring major non-elective intervention
Hepatic		
$> 2.5 – 5.0 \times$ ULN	$> 5.0 – 20.0 \times$ ULN	$> 20.0 \times$ ULN
$> 1.5 – 3.0 \times$ ULN	$> 3.0 – 10.0 \times$ ULN	$> 10.0 \times$ ULN
$\geq 3 – < 6$ mg/100 mL	$\geq 6 – < 15$ mg/100 mL	≥ 15 mg/100 mL
$\geq 2.5 – 5.0 \times$ ULN	$> 5.0 – 20.0 \times$ ULN	$> 20.0 \times$ ULN

Table 1 Common Toxicity Criteria (CTC) *Continued*

		Grade
Adverse Event	**0**	**1**
Hepatic		
Hepatic enlargement	absent	—
Note: Grade Hepatic enlargement only for treatment related adverse event including Veno-occlusive Disease.		
Hypoalbuminemia	WNL	$<$ LLN – 3 g/dL
Liver dysfunction/ failure (clinical)	normal	—
Portal vein flow	normal	—
SGOT (AST) (serum glutamic pyruvic transaminase)	WNL	$>$ ULN – 2.5 $\times$ ULN
SGPT (ALT) (serum glutamic pyruvic transaminase)	WNL	$>$ ULN – 2.5 $\times$ ULN
Hepatic —Other (Specify, _____)	none	mild
Infection/Febrile Neutropenia		
Catheter-related infection	none	mild, no active treatment
Febrile neutropenia (fever of unknown origin without clinically or microbiologically documented infection) (ANC $<$ 1.0 $\times$ 10^9/L, fever $\geq$ 38.5°C)	none	—
Note: Hypothermia instead of fever may be associated with neutropenia and is graded here.		

2	Grade 3	4
	Hepatic	
—	present	—
$\geq 2 - < 3$ g/dL	< 2 g/dL	—
—	asterixis	encephalopathy or coma
decreased portal vein flow	reversal/retrograde portal vein flow	—
$\geq 2.5 - 5.0 \times$ ULN	$> 5.0 - 20.0 \times$ ULN	$> 20.0 \times$ ULN
$\geq 2.5 - 5.0 \times$ ULN	$> 5.0 - 20.0 \times$ ULN	$> 20.0 \times$ ULN
moderate	severe	life-threatening or disabling
	Infection/Febrile Neutropenia	
moderate, localized infection, requiring local or oral treatment	severe, systemic infection, requiring IV antibiotic or antifungal treatment or hospitalization	life-threatening sepsis (e.g., septic shock)
—	present	life-threatening sepsis (e.g., septic shock)

Table 1 Common Toxicity Criteria (CTC) *Continued*

Adverse Event	Grade 0	Grade 1
Infection/Febrile Neutropenia		
Infection (documented clinically or micro-biologically) with grade 3 or 4 neutropenia (ANC $< 1.0 \times 10^9$/L)	none	—
Notes: Hypothermia instead of fever may be associated with neutropenia and is graded here. In the absence of documented infection grade 3 or 4 neutropenia with fever is graded as Febrile neutropenia.		
Infection with unknown ANC	none	—
Note: This adverse event criterion is used in the rare case when ANC is unknown.		
Infection without neutropenia	none	mild, no active treatment or oral treatment
Wound-infection is graded in the DERMATOLOGY/SKIN category.		
Infection/Febrile Neutropenia - Other (Specify, _____)	none	mild
Lymphatics		
Lymphatics	normal	mild lymphedema
Lymphatics - Other (Specify, _____)	none	mild

	Grade	
2	**3**	**4**
Infection/Febrile Neutropenia		
—	present	life-threatening sepsis (e.g., septic shock)
—	present	life-threatening sepsis (e.g., septic shock)
moderate, localized infection, requiring local antibiotic or antifungal treatment, or hospitalization	severe, systemic infection, requiring IV	life-threatening sepsis (e.g., septic shock)
moderate	severe	life-threatening or disabling
Lymphatics		
moderate lymphedema requiring compression; lymphocyst	severe lymphedema limiting function; lymphocyst requiring surgery	severe lymphedema limiting function with ulceration
moderate	severe	life-threatening or disabling

Table 1 Common Toxicity Criteria (CTC) *Continued*

Adverse Event	Grade 0	Grade 1
Metabolic/Laboratory		
Acidosis (metabolic or respiratory)	normal	pH < normal, but ≤ 7.3
Alkalosis (metabolic or respiratory)	normal	pH > normal, but ≤ 7.5
Amylase	WNL	> ULN – 1.5 × ULN
Bicarbonate	WNL	< LLN – 16 mEq/dL
CPK (creatine phosphokinase)	WNL	> ULN – 2.5 × ULN
Hypercalcemia	WNL	> ULN – 11.5 mg/dL > ULN – 2.9 mmol/L
Hypercholesterolemia	WNL	> ULN – 300 mg/dL > ULN – 7.75 mmol/L
Hyperglycemia	WNL	> ULN – 160 mg/dL > ULN - 8.9 mmol/L
Hyperkalemia	WNL	> ULN - 5.5 mmol/L
Hypermagnesemia	WNL	> ULN - 3.0 mg/dL > ULN – 1.23 mmol/L
Hypernatremia	WNL	> ULN – 150 mmol/L
Hypertriglyceridemia	WNL	> ULN – 2.5 × ULN
Hyperuricemia	WNL	> ULN – ≤ 10 mg/dL ≤ 0.59 mmol/L without physiologic consequences
Hypocalcemia	WNL	< LLN – 8.0 mg/dL < LLN – 2.0 mmol/L
Hypoglycemia	WNL	< LLN – 55 mg/dL < LLN – 3.0 mmol/L

2	3	4
	Grade	
	Metabolic/Laboratory	
—	pH < 7.3	pH < 7.3 with life-threatening physiologic consequences
—	pH > 7.5	pH > 7.5 with life-threatening physiologic consequences
> 1.5 – 2.0 × ULN	> 2.0 – 5.0 × ULN	> 5.0 × ULN
11 – 15 mEq/dL	8 – 10 mEq/dL	> 8 mEq/dL
> 2.5 – 5 × ULN	> 5 – 10 × ULN	> 10 × ULN
> 11.5 – 12.5 mg/dL > 2.9 – 3.1 mmol/L	> 12.5 – 13.5 mg/dL > 3.1 – 3.4 mmol/L	> 13.5 mg/dL > 3.4 mmol/L
> 300 – 400 mg/dL > 7.75 – 10.34 mmol/L	> 400 – 500 mg/dL > 10.34 – 12.92 mmol/L	> 500 mg/dL > 12.92 mmol/L
> 160 – 250 mg/dL > 8.9 – 13.9 mmol/L	> 250 – 500 mg/dL > 13.9 – 27.8 mmol/L	> 500 mg/dL > 27.8 mmol/L or acidosis
> 5.5 – 6.0 mmol/L	> 6.0 – 7.0 mmol/L	> 7.0 mmol/L
—	> 3.0 – 8.0 mg/dL > 1.23 – 3.30 mmol/L	> 8.0 mg/dL > 3.30 mmol/L
> 150 – 155 mmol/L	> 155 – 160 mmol/L	> 160 mmol/L
> 2.5 – 5.0 × ULN	> 5.0 – 10 × ULN	> 10 × ULN
—	> ULN – ≤ 10 mg/dL ≤ 0.59 mmol/L with physiologic consequences	> 10 mg/dL > 0.59 mmol/L
7.0 – < 8.0 mg/dL 1.75 – < 2.0 mmol/L	6.0 – < 7.0 mg/dL 1.5 – < 1.75 mmol/L	< 6.0 mg/dL < 1.5 mmol/L
40 – < 55 mg/dL 2.2 – < 3.0 mmol/L	30 – < 40 mg/dL 1.7 – < 2.2 mmol/L	< 3.0 mg/dL < 1.7 mmol/L

Table 1 Common Toxicity Criteria (CTC) *Continued*

Adverse Event	Grade 0	Grade 1
Metabolic/Laboratory		
Hypokalemia	WNL	< LLN – 3.0 mmol/L
Hypomagnesemia	WNL	< LLN – 1.2 mg/dL < LLN – 0.5 mmol/L
Hyponatremia	WNL	< LLN – 130 mmol/L
Hypophosphatemia	WNL	< LLN – 2.5 mg/dL < LLN – 0.8 mmol/L
Hypothyroidism is graded in the ENDOCRINE category.		
Lipase	WNL	> ULN – 1.5 × ULN
Metabolic/Laboratory—Other (Specify, _____)	none	mild
Musculoskeletal		
Arthralgia is graded in the PAIN category.		
Arthritis	none	mild pain with inflammation, erythema or joint swelling but not interfering with function
Muscle weakness (not due to neuropathy)	normal	asymptomatic with weakness on physical exam
Myalgia [tenderness or pain in muscles] is graded in the PAIN category.		
Myositis (inflammation/damage of muscle)	none	mild pain, not interfering with function

Note: Myositis implies muscle damage (i.e., elevated CPK).

	Grade	
2	**3**	**4**
Metabolic/Laboratory		
—	2.5 – < 3.0 mmol/L	< 2.5 mmol/L
0.9 – < 1.2 mg/dL 0.4 – < 0.5 mmol/L	0.7 – < 0.9 mg/dL 0.3 – < 0.4 mmol/L	< 0.7 mg/dL < 0.3 mmol/L
—	120 – < 130 mmol/L	< 120 mmol/L
≥ 2.0 – < 1.2 mg/dL ≥ 0.6 – < 0.8 mmol/L	≥ 1.0 – < 2.0 mg/dL ≥ 0.3 – < 0.6 mmol/L	< 1.0 mg/dL < 0.3 mmol/L
> 1.5 – 2.0 × ULN	> 2.0 – 5.0 × ULN	> 5.0 × ULN
moderate	severe	life-threatening or disabling
Musculoskeletal		
moderate pain with inflammation, erythema, or joint swelling interfering with function, but not interfering with activities of daily living	severe pain with inflammation, erythema, or joint swelling and interfering with activities of daily living	disabling
symptomatic and interfering with function, but not interfering with activities of daily living	symptomatic and interfering with activities of daily living	bedridden or disabling
pain interfering with function, but not interfering with activities of daily living	pain interfering with function and interfering with activities of daily living	bedridden or disabling

Table 1 Common Toxicity Criteria (CTC) *Continued*

		Grade
Adverse Event	**0**	**1**
Muskuloskeletal		
Osteonecrosis (avascular necrosis)	none	asymptomatic and detected by imaging only
Musculoskeletal—Other (Specify, _____)	none	mild
Neurology		
Aphasia, receptive and/or expressive, is graded under Speech impairment in the NEUROLOGY category.		
Arachnoiditis/ meningismus/ radiculitis	absent	mild pain not interfering with function
Ataxia (incoordination)	normal	asymptomatic but abnormal on physical exam, and not interfering with function
CNS cerebrovascular ischemia	none	—
CNS hemorrhage/bleeding is graded in the HEMORRHAGE category.		
cognitive disturbance/ learning problems *For pediatric patients, systolic BP 65 mmHg or less in infants up to 1 year old and 70 mmHg or less in children older than 1 year of age, use two successive or three measurements in 24 hours.*	*none*	*cognitive disability; not interfering with work/ school performance; preservation of intelligence*

Grade		
2	**3**	**4**
Muskuloskeletal		
symptomatic and interfering with function, but not interfering with activities of daily living	symptomatic and interfering with activities of daily living	symptomatic or disabling;
moderate	severe	life-threatening or disabling
Neurology		
moderate pain interfering with function, but not interfering with activities of daily living	severe pain interfering with activities of daily living	unable to function or perform activities of daily living; bedridden; paraplegia
mild symptoms interfering with function, but not interfering with activities of daily living	moderate symptoms interfering with activities of daily living	bedridden or disabling
—	transient ischemic event or attack (TIA)	permanent event (e.g., cerebral vascular accident)
cognitive disability; interfering with work/ school performance; decline of 1 SD (Standard Deviation) or loss of development milestones	*cognitive disability; resulting in significant impairment of work/school performance; cognitive decline > 2 SD (Standard deviation)*	*inability to work/frank mental retardation*

Table 1 Common Toxicity Criteria (CTC) *Continued*

	Grade	
Adverse Event	**0**	**1**
Neurology		
Confusion	normal	confusion or disorientation or attention deficit of brief duration; resolves spontaneously with no sequelae
Cranial neuropathy is graded in the NEUROLOGY category as Neuropathy-cranial.		
Delusions	normal	—
Depressed level of consciousness	normal	somnolence or sedation not interfering with function
Note: Syncope (fainting) is graded in the NEUROLOGY category.		
Dizziness/ lightheadedness	none	not interfering with function
Dysphasia, receptive and/or expressive, is graded under Speech impairment in the NEUROLOGY category.		
Extrapyramidal/ involuntary movement/restlessness	none	mild involuntary movements not interfering with function
Hallucinations	normal	—
Headache is graded in the PAIN category.		
Insomnia	normal	occasional difficulty sleeping not interfering with function
Note: This adverse event is graded when insomnia is related to treatment. If pain or other symptoms interfere with sleep do *not* grade as insomnia.		

	Grade	
2	**3**	**4**
	Neurology	
confusion or disorientation or attention deficit interfering with function, but not interfering with activities of daily living	confusion or delirium interfering with activities of daily living	harmful to others or self; requiring hospitalization
—	present	toxic psychosis
somnolence or sedation interfering with function, but not interfering with activities of daily living	obtundation or stupor; difficult to arouse; interfering with activities of daily living	coma
interfering with function, but not interfering with activities of daily living	interfering with activities of daily living	bedridden or disabling
moderate involuntary movements interfering with function, but not interfering with activities of daily living	severe involuntary movements or torticollis interfering with activities of daily living	bedridden or disabling
—	present	toxic psychosis
difficulty sleeping interfering with function, but not interfering with activities of daily living	frequent difficulty sleeping, interfering with activities of daily living	—

Table 1 Common Toxicity Criteria (CTC) *Continued*

Adverse Event	Grade 0	1
Neurology		
Irritability (children < 3 years of age)	*normal*	*mild; easily consolable*
Leukoencephalopathy associated radiological findings	none	mild increase in SAS (subarachnoid space) and/or mild ventriculomegaly; and/or small (+/− multiple) focal T2 hyperintensities, involving periventricular white matter or < 1/3 of susceptible areas of cerebrum
Memory loss	normal	memory loss not interfering with function
Mood alteration-anxiety, agitation	normal	mild mood alteration not interfering with function
Mood alteration-depression	normal	mild mood alteration not interfering with function
Mood alteration-euphoria	normal	mild mood alteration not interfering with function
Neuropathic pain is graded in the PAIN category.		
Neuropathy-cranial	absent	—

	Grade	
2	**3**	**4**
Neurology		
moderate; requiring increased attention	*severe; inconsolable*	—
moderate increase in SAS; and/or moderate ventriculomegaly; and/or focal T2 hyperintensities extending into centrum ovale; or involving 1/3 to 2/3 of susceptible areas of cerebrum	severe increase in SAS; severe ventriculomegaly; near total white matter T2 hyperintensities or diffuse low attenuation (CT); focal white matter necrosis (cystic)	severe increase in SAS; severe ventriculomegaly; diffuse low attenuation with calcification (CT); diffuse white matter necrosis (MRI)
memory loss interfering with function, but not interfering with activities of daily living	memory loss interfering with activities of daily living	amnesia
moderate mood alteration interfering with function, but not interfering with activities of daily living	severe mood alteration interfering with activities of daily living	suicidal ideation or danger to self
moderate mood alteration interfering with function, but not interfering with activities of daily living	severe mood alteration interfering with activities of daily living	suicidal ideation or danger to self
moderate mood alteration interfering with function, but not interfering with activities of daily living	severe mood alteration interfering with activities of daily living	danger to self
present, not interfering with activities of daily living	present, interfering with activities of daily living	life-threatening, disabling

Table 1 Common Toxicity Criteria (CTC) *Continued*

	Grade	
Adverse Event	**0**	**1**
Neurology		
Neuropathy-motor	normal	subjective weakness but no objective findings
Neuropathy-sensory	normal	loss of deep tendon reflexes or paresthesia (including tingling) but not interfering with function
Nystagmus	absent	present
Personality/behavioral	normal	change, but not disruptive to patient or family
Pyramidal tract dysfunction (e.g., ↑ tone, hyperreflexia, positive Babinski, ↓ fine motor coordination)	normal	asymptomatic with abnormality on physical examination
Seizure(s)	none	—
Speech impairment (e.g., dysphasia or aphasia)	normal	—
Syncope (fainting)	absent	—
Tremor	none	mild and brief or intermittent but not interfering with function

	Grade	
2	**3**	**4**
Neurology		
mild objective weakness interfering with function, but not interfering with activities of daily living	objective weakness interfering with activities of daily living	paralysis
objective sensory loss or paresthesia (including tingling), interfering with function, but not interfering with activities of daily living	sensory loss or paresthesia interfering with activities of daily living	permanent sensory loss that interferes with function
—	—	—
disruptive to patient or family	disruptive to patient and family; requiring mental health intervention	harmful to others or self; requiring hospitalization
symptomatic or interfering with function but not interfering with activities of daily living	interfering with activities of daily living	bedridden or disabling; paralysis
seizure(s) self-limited and consciousness is preserved	seizure(s) in which consciousness is altered	seizures of any type which are prolonged, repetitive, or difficult to control (e.g., status epilepticus, intractable epilepsy)
awareness of receptive or expressive dysphasia, not impairing ability to communicate	receptive or expressive dysphasia, impairing ability to communicate	inability to communicate
—	present	—
moderate tremor interfering with function, but not interfering with activities of daily living	severe tremor interfering with activities of daily living	—

Table 1 Common Toxicity Criteria (CTC) *Continued*

Adverse Event	Grade 0	Grade 1
Neurology		
Vertigo	none	not interfering with function
Neurology—Other (Specify, _____)	none	mild
Ocular/Visual		
Cataract	none	asymptomatic
Conjunctivitis	none	abnormal ophthalmologic changes, but asymptomatic or symptomatic without visual impairment (i.e., pain and irritation)
Dry eye	normal	mild, not requiring treatment
Glaucoma	none	increase in intraocular pressure but no visual loss
Keratitis (corneal inflammation/corneal ulceration)	none	abnormal ophthalmologic changes but asymptomatic or symptomatic without visual impairment (i.e., pain and irritation)
Tearing (watery eyes)	none	mild: not interfering with function

	Grade	
2	**3**	**4**
	Neurology	
interfering with function, but not interfering with activities of daily living	interfering with activities of daily living	bedridden or disabling
moderate	severe	life-threatening or disabling
	Ocular/Visual	
symptomatic, partial visual loss	symptomatic, visual loss requiring treatment or interfering with function	—
symptomatic and interfering with function, but not interfering with activities of daily living	symptomatic and interfering with activities of daily living	—
moderate or requiring artificial tears	—	—
increase in intraocular pressure with retinal changes	visual impairment	unilateral or bilateral loss of vision (blindness)
symptomatic and interfering with function, but not interfering with activities of daily living	symptomatic and interfering with activities of daily living	unilateral or bilateral loss of vision (blindness)
moderate: interfering with function, but not interfering with activities of daily living	interfering with activities of daily living	—

Table 1 Common Toxicity Criteria (CTC) *Continued*

Adverse Event	Grade 0	1
Ocular/Visual		
Vision-blurred vision	normal	—
Vision-double vision (diplopia)	normal	—
Vision-flashing lights/ floaters	normal	mild, not interfering with function
Vision-night blindness (nyctalopia)	normal	abnormal electro-retinography but asymptomatic
Vision-photophobia	normal	—
Ocular/Visual—Other (Specify, _____)	normal	mild
Pain		
Abdominal pain or cramping	none	mild pain not interfering with function
Arthralgia (joint pain)	none	mild pain not interfering with function

	Grade	
2	**3**	**4**
Ocular/Visual		
symptomatic and interfering with function, but not interfering with activities of daily living	symptomatic and interfering with activities of daily living	—
symptomatic and interfering with function, but not interfering with activities of daily living	symptomatic and interfering with activities of daily living	—
symptomatic and interfering with function, but not interfering with activities of daily living	symptomatic and interfering with activities of daily living	—
symptomatic and interfering with function, but not interfering with activities of daily living	symptomatic and interfering with activities of daily living	—
symptomatic and interfering with function, but not interfering with activities of daily living	symptomatic and interfering with activities of daily living	—
moderate	severe	unilateral or bilateral loss of vision (blindness)
Pain		
moderate pain: pain or analgesics interfering with function, but not interfering with activities of daily living	severe pain: pain or analgesics severely interfering with activities of daily living	disabling
moderate pain: pain or analgesics interfering with function, but not interfering with activities of daily living	severe pain: pain or analgesics severely interfering with activities of daily living	disabling

Table 1 Common Toxicity Criteria (CTC) *Continued*

Adverse Event	0	Grade 1
Pain		
Arthritis (joint pain with clinical signs of inflammation) is graded in the MUSCULOSKELETAL category.		
Bone pain	none	mild pain not interfering with function
Chest pain (non-cardiac and nonpleuritic)	none	mild pain not interfering with function
Dysmenorrhea	none	mild pain not interfering with function
Dyspareunia	none	mild pain not interfering with function
Dysuria is graded in the RENAL/GENITOURINARY category.		
Earache (otalgia)	none	mild pain not interfering with function
Headache	none	mild pain not interfering with function
Hepatic pain	none	mild pain not interfering with function

	Grade	
2	**3**	**4**
	Pain	
moderate pain: pain or analgesics interfering with function, but not interfering with activities of daily living	severe pain: pain or analgesics severely interfering with activities of daily living	disabling
moderate pain: pain or analgesics interfering with function, but not interfering with activities of daily living	severe pain: pain or analgesics severely interfering with activities of daily living	disabling
moderate pain: pain or analgesics interfering with function, but not interfering with activities of daily living	severe pain: pain or analgesics severely interfering with activities of daily living	disabling
moderate pain interfering with sexual activity	severe pain preventing sexual activity	—
moderate pain: pain or analgesics interfering with function, but not interfering with activities of daily living	severe pain: pain or analgesics severely interfering with activities of daily living	disabling
moderate pain: pain or analgesics interfering with function, but not interfering with activities of daily living	severe pain: pain or analgesics severely interfering with activities of daily living	disabling
moderate pain: pain or analgesics interfering with function, but not interfering with activities of daily living	severe pain: pain or analgesics severely interfering with activities of daily living	disabling

Table 1 Common Toxicity Criteria (CTC) *Continued*

		Grade
Adverse Event	**0**	**1**
Pain		
Myalgia (muscle pain)	none	mild pain not interfering with function
Neuropathic pain (e.g., jaw pain, neurologic pain, phantom limb pain, post-infectious neuralgia, or painful neuropathies)	none	mild pain not interfering with function
Pain due to radiation	none	mild pain not interfering with function
Pelvic pain	none	mild pain not interfering with function
Pleuritic pain	none	mild pain not interfering with function
Rectal or perirectal pain (proctalgia)	none	mild pain not interfering with function
Tumor pain (onset or exacerbation of tumor pain due to treatment)	none	mild pain not interfering with function
Tumor flare is graded in the SYNDROME category.		

	Grade	
2	**3**	**4**
	Pain	
moderate pain: pain or analgesics interfering with function, but not interfering with activities of daily living	severe pain: pain or analgesics severely interfering with activities of daily living	disabling
moderate pain: pain or analgesics interfering with function, but not interfering with activities of daily living	severe pain: pain or analgesics severely interfering with activities of daily living	disabling
moderate pain: pain or analgesics interfering with function, but not interfering with activities of daily living	severe pain: pain or analgesics severely interfering with activities of daily living	disabling
moderate pain: pain or analgesics interfering with function, but not interfering with activities of daily living	severe pain: pain or analgesics severely interfering with activities of daily living	disabling
moderate pain: pain or analgesics interfering with function, but not interfering with activities of daily living	severe pain: pain or analgesics severely interfering with activities of daily living	disabling
moderate pain: pain or analgesics interfering with function, but not interfering with activities of daily living	severe pain: pain or analgesics severely interfering with activities of daily living	disabling
moderate pain: pain or analgesics interfering with function, but not interfering with activities of daily living	severe pain: pain or analgesics severely interfering with activities of daily living	disabling

Table 1 Common Toxicity Criteria (CTC) *Continued*

Adverse Event	Grade 0	Grade 1
Pain		
Pain - Other (Specify, _____)	none	mild
Pulmonary		
Adult Respiratory Distress Syndrome (ARDS)	absent	—
Apnea	none	—
Carbon monoxide diffusion capacity (DL_{CO})	$\geq 90\%$ of pretreatment or normal value	$\geq 75 - < 90\%$ of pretreatment or normal value
Cough	absent	mild, relieved by nonprescription medication
Dyspnea (shortness of breath)	normal	—
FEV_1	$\geq 90\%$ of pretreatment or normal value	$\geq 75 - < 90\%$ of pretreatment or normal value
Hiccoughs (hiccups, singultus)	none	mild, not requiring treatment
Hypoxia	normal	—
Pleural effusion (non-malignant)	none	asymptomatic and not requiring treatment
Pleuritic pain is graded in the PAIN category.		

	Grade	
2	**3**	**4**
Pain		
moderate	severe	disabling
Pulmonary		
—	—	present
—	present	requiring intubation
≥ 50 – < 75% of pretreatment or normal value	≥ 25 – < 50% of pretreatment or normal value	< 25% of pretreatment or normal value
requiring narcotic antitussive	severe cough or coughing spasms, poorly controlled or unresponsive to treatment	—
dyspnea on exertion	dyspnea at normal level of activity	dyspnea at rest or requiring ventilator support
≥ 50 – < 75% of pretreatment or normal value	≥ 25 – < 50% of pretreatment or normal value	< 25% of pretreatment or normal value
moderate, requiring treatment	severe, prolonged, and refractory to treatment	—
decreased O_2 saturation with exercise	decreased O_2 saturation at rest, requiring supplemental oxygen	decreased O_2 saturation, requiring pressure support (CPAP) or assisted ventilation
symptomatic, requiring diuretics	symptomatic, requiring O_2 or therapeutic thoracentesis	life-threatening (e.g., requiring intubation)

Table 1 Common Toxicity Criteria (CTC) *Continued*

Adverse Event	Grade 0	Grade 1
Pulmonary		
Pneumonitis/pulmonary infiltrates	none	radiographic changes but asymptomatic or symptoms not requiring steroids
Pneumothorax	none	no intervention required
Pulmonary embolism is graded as Thrombosis/embolism in the CARDIOVASCULAR (GENERAL) category.		
Pulmonary fibrosis	none	radiographic changes, but asymptomatic or symptoms not requiring steroids
Voice changes/stridor/larynx (e.g., hoarseness, loss of voice, laryngitis)	normal	mild or intermittent hoarseness
Notes: Cough from radiation is graded as cough in the PULMONARY category. Radiation-related hemoptysis from larynx/pharynx is graded as grade 4 Mucositis due to radiation in the GASTROINTESTINAL category. Radiation-related hemoptysis from the thoracic cavity is graded as grade 4 Hemoptysis in the HEMORRHAGE category.		
Pulmonary–Other (Specify, _____)	none	mild
Renal/Genitourinary		
Bladder spasms	absent	mild symptoms, not requiring intervention
Creatinine	WNL	$> ULN - 1.5 \times ULN$
Note: Adjust to age-appropriate levels for pediatric patients.		
Dysuria (painful urination)	none	mild symptoms requiring no intervention

	Grade	
2	**3**	**4**
	Pulmonary	
radiographic changes and requiring steroids or diuretics	radiographic changes and requiring oxygen	radiographic changes and requiring assisted ventilation
chest tube required	sclerosis or surgery required	life-threatening
requiring steroids or diuretics	requiring oxygen	requiring assisted ventilation
persistent hoarseness, but able to vocalize; may have mild to moderate edema	whispered speech, not able to vocalize; may have marked edema	marked dyspnea/stridor requiring tracheostomy or intubation
moderate	severe	life-threatening or disabling
	Renal/Genitourinary	
symptoms requiring antispasmodic	severe symptoms requiring narcotic	—
> 1.5 – 3.0 × ULN	> 3.0 – 6.0 × ULN	> 6.0 × ULN
symptoms relieved with therapy	symptoms not relieved despite therapy	—

Table 1 Common Toxicity Criteria (CTC) *Continued*

Adverse Event	Grade 0	Grade 1
Renal/Genitourinary		
Fistula or GU fistula (e.g., vaginal, vesicovaginal)	none	—
Hemoglobinuria	—	present
Hematuria (in the absence of vaginal bleeding) is graded in the HEMORRHAGE category.		
Incontinence	none	with coughing, sneezing, etc.
Operative injury to bladder and/or ureter	none	—
Proteinuria	normal or < 0.15 g/ 24 hours	1+ or 0.15 – 1.0 g/ 24 hours
Note: If there is an inconsistency between absolute value and dip stick reading, use the absolute value for grading.		
Renal failure	none	—
Ureteral obstruction	none	unilateral, not requiring surgery
Urinary electrolyte wasting (e.g., Fanconi's syndrome, renal tubular acidosis)	none	asymptomatic, not requiring treatment
Urinary frequency/ urgency	normal	increase in frequency or nocturia up to 2 × normal

	Grade	
2	3	4
Renal/Genitourinary		
—	requiring intervention	requiring surgery
—	—	—
spontaneous, some control	no control (in the absence of fistula)	—
injury of bladder with primary repair	sepsis, fistula, or obstruction requiring secondary surgery; loss of one kidney; injury requiring anastomosis or re-implantation	septic obstruction of both kidneys or vesicovaginal fistula requiring diversion
2+ to 3+ or 1.0 – 3.5 g/ 24 hours	4+ or > 3.5 g/24 hours	nephrotic syndrome
—	requiring dialysis, but reversible	requiring dialysis and irreversible
—	bilateral, not requiring surgery	stent, nephrostomy tube, or surgery
mild, reversible and manageable with oral replacement	reversible but requiring IV replacement	irreversible, requiring continued replacement
increase > 2 × normal but < hourly	hourly or more with urgency, or requiring catheter	—

Table 1 Common Toxicity Criteria (CTC) *Continued*

Adverse Event	Grade 0	Grade 1
Renal/Genitourinary		
Urinary retention	normal	hesitancy or dribbling, but no significant residual urine; retention occurring during the immediate postoperative period
Urine color change (not related to other dietary or physiologic cause e.g., bilirubin, concentrated urine, hematuria)	normal	asymptomatic, change in urine color
Vaginal bleeding is graded in the HEMORRHAGE category.		
Vaginitis (not due to infection)	none	mild, not requiring treatment
Renal/Genitourinary—Other (Specify, ____)	none	mild
Secondary Malignancy		
Secondary Malignancy—Other (Specify type, ____) excludes metastasis from initial primary	none	—
Sexual/Reproductive Function		
Dyspareunia is graded in the PAIN category.		
Dysmenorrhea is graded in the PAIN category.		
Erectile impotence	normal	mild (erections impaired but satisfactory)
Female sterility	normal	—

	Grade	
2	**3**	**4**
Renal/Genitourinary		
hesitancy requiring medication or occasional in/out catheterization (< 4 × per week), or operative bladder atony requiring indwelling catheter beyond immediate postoperative period but for < 6 weeks	requiring frequent in/out catheterization (≥ 4 × per week) or urological intervention (e.g., TURP, suprapubic tube, urethrotomy)	bladder rupture
—	—	—
moderate, relieved with treatment	severe, not relieved with treatment, or ulceration not requiring surgery	ulceration requiring surgery
moderate	severe	life-threatening or disabling
Secondary Malignancy		
—	—	present
Sexual/Reproductive Function		
moderate (erections impaired, unsatisfactory for intercourse)	no erections	—
—	sterile	—

Table 1 Common Toxicity Criteria (CTC) *Continued*

		Grade
Adverse Event	**0**	**1**
Sexual/Reproductive Function		
Feminization of male is graded in the ENDOCRINE category.		
Irregular menses (change from baseline)	normal	occasionally irregular or lengthened interval, but continuing menstrual cycles
Libido	normal	decrease in interest
Male infertility	—	—
Masculinization of female is graded in the ENDOCRINE category.		
Vaginal dryness	normal	mild
Sexual/Reproductive Function - Other (Specify, _____)	none	mild
Syndromes (not included in previous categories)		
Acute vascular leak syndrome is graded in the CARDIOVASCULAR (GENERAL) category.		
ARDS (Adult Respiratory Distress Syndrome) is graded in the PULMONARY category.		
Autoimmune reactions are graded in the ALLERGY/IMMUNOLOGY category.		
DIC (disseminated intravascular coagulation) is graded in the COAGULATION category.		
Fanconi's syndrome is graded as Urinary electrolyte wasting in the RENAL/GENITOURINARY category.		
Renal tubular acidosis is graded as Urinary electrolyte wasting in the RENAL/GENITOURINARY category.		
Stevens-Johnson syndrome (erythema multiforme) is graded in the DERMATOLOGY/SKIN category.		
SIADH (syndrome of inappropriate antidiuretic hormone) is graded in the ENDOCRINE category.		

	Grade	
2	**3**	**4**
Sexual/Reproductive Function		
very irregular, but continuing menstrual cycles	persistent amenorrhea	—
severe loss of interest	—	—
oligospermia (low sperm count)	azoospermia (no sperm)	—
requiring treatment and/or interfering with sexual function, dyspareunia	—	—
moderate	severe	disabling
Syndromes (not included in previous categories)		

Table 1 Common Toxicity Criteria (CTC) *Continued*

Adverse Event	0	Grade 1
Syndromes (not included in previous categories)		
Thrombotic microangiopathy (e.g., thrombotic thrombocytopenic purpura/TTP or hemolytic uremic syndrome/HUS) is graded in the COAGULATION category.		
Tumor flare	none	mild pain not interfering with function
Note: Tumor flare is characterized by a constellation of symptoms and signs in direct relation to initiation of therapy (e.g., anti-estrogens/androgens or additional hormones). The symptoms/signs include tumor pain, inflammation of visible tumor, hypercalcemia, diffuse bone pain, and other electrolyte disturbances.		
Tumor lysis syndrome	absent	—
Urinary electrolyte wasting (e.g., Fanconi's syndrome, renal tubular acidosis) is graded in the RENAL/GENITOURINARY category.		
Syndromes - Other (Specify, _____)	none	mild

	Grade	
2	3	4
Syndromes (not included in previous categories)		
moderate pain; pain or analgesics interfering with function, but not interfering with activities of daily living	severe pain; pain or analgesics interfering with function and interfering with activities of daily living	disabling
—	present	—
moderate	severe	life-threatening or disabling

Table 2 Standardized Nursing Care Plan for Patient
Experiencing Bone Marrow Depression

Nursing Diagnosis	Expected Outcomes
I. A. *Potential for altered health maintenance*	I. A. Pt will manage self-care as evidenced by verbal recall or return demonstration of instructions for self-assessment of oral temperature; examination of skin and mucous membranes; signs and symptoms of infection and bleeding; measures to avoid exposure to infection; measures to avoid injury and bleeding; and when and how to notify the health care provider
B. *Potential for noncompliance with self-care activities*	B. Pt and significant other will comply with prescribed measures 90% of the time
C. *Knowledge deficit related to purpose and self-administration techniques of cytokine growth factors, which may be given to prevent complications of febrile neutropenia, anemia, or bleeding*	C. Pt and significant other will verbally describe and demonstrate technique for administration of growth factors if ordered

---

Nursing Intervention

I.   A. 1. Assess baseline knowledge, learning style, level of anxiety of pt and
              significant other
         2. Develop and implement teaching plan
             a. Purpose and goal of chemotherapy
             b. Specific drugs
                 1) mechanism of action
                 2) potential side effects, including bone marrow suppression as
                     appropriate
             c. Self-care measures
                 1) assessment and care of skin, oral mucosa to prevent infection,
                     trauma
                 2) assessment of temperature BID, or if feels as if fever, and
                     instructions to call health care provider if temperature is over
                     101°F (38.5°C)
                 3) signs and symptoms of infection (fever, sore throat, cough,
                     painful urination)
                 4) signs and symptoms of bleeding (nose or gum bleeding,
                     capillary or large "black and blues")
                 5) measures to minimize exposure to infection and trauma as des-
                     cribed in NCI booklet *Chemotherapy and You: A Guide to Self-Help*
             d. Provide written information to reinforce teaching, such as the
                 booklet above, free from the NCI

     B. 1. Reinforce teaching prior to treatment as nurse does prechemo
             assessment and prior to pt leaving clinic or hospital after treatment
             administration
         2. Evaluate compliance through telephone call to pt following treatment
             or discharge or visiting nurse home visit
         3. If pt or significant other is having difficulty with managing self-care
             activities, consider visiting nurse referral or hospitalization if pt is
             neutropenic or thrombocytopenic and unable to safely care for self

     C. 1. Provide teaching regarding side effects and administration techniques
             using video, pt education booklets, and demonstration/return
             demonstration
         2. If unable to manage administration, contact community nursing
             agencies
         3. Pt/family teaching materials available through the pharmaceutical
             companies that make cytokine growth factors

Table 2 Standardized Nursing Care Plan for Patient
Experiencing Bone Marrow Depression *Continued*

Nursing Diagnosis	Expected Outcomes
II. *Potential for altered nutrition: less than body requirements*	II. A. Pt will maintain within 5% of pretreatment weight B. Recovery from nadir approximates expected time based on specific chemotherapy agents
III. *Potential for injury: infection and bleeding related to bone marrow depression*	III. A. Pt will remain free of infection, bleeding, and tissue hypoxia B. Pt will experience minimal complications of bone marrow suppression as evidenced by return to normal temperature and neutrophil count and absence of major bleeding

---

Nursing Intervention

II. A. Assess food preferences
   B. Encourage foods high in proteins, calories, iron, and folic acid
   C. Discourage excessive alcohol intake
   D. Review dietary instructions with pt and person responsible for preparing food
   E. Review teaching material with pt and family from NCI booklet *Eating Hints* for pts receiving chemotherapy, a free publication

---

III. A. Assess potential for injury related to bone marrow depression
       1. Expected nadir from specific agents administered, nadir from prior treatment cycle if appropriate
       2. Major life stressors and coping ability
       3. Sexual history and self-care habits re: hygiene
       4. Sleep pattern
       5. Elimination pattern
       6. Nutritional pattern
       7. History and physical exam
          a. Symptoms of infection: fever, pain (swallowing, with elimination, etc.), erythema, presence of exudate
          b. Symptoms of bleeding: dizziness, presence of blood in excreta
          c. Symptoms of anemia: fatigue, dyspnea on exertion, angina
          d. Skin, mucous membranes: are they intact, color, evidence of petechiae or ecchymoses, exudate
          e. Breath sounds, pulmonary exam
          f. CNS exam
          g. Laboratory data: complete blood count, WBC differential, absolute neutrophil count
    B. Institute neutropenic precautions for absolute neutrophil count $< 500/mm^3$
       1. Protect pt from exposure to microorganisms
          a. Provide private room if possible
          b. Place sign on door requiring *all* persons who enter to wash their hands meticulously prior to entering the room, that persons with colds or infections should not enter, and that no flowers, fresh fruits, or vegetables should be brought into the room
          c. Place card in nursing cardex instructing that *no* intramuscular injections, rectal temperatures, or medications should be administered PR
          d. Plan scrupulous hygiene with pt for oral care, daily bath, and meticulous perineal hygiene
          e. Inspect all intravenous sites and change dressings using asceptic technique; sites should be changed every 48 hours or earlier if there is any indication of phlebitis

Table 2 Standardized Nursing Care Plan for Patient
           Experiencing Bone Marrow Depression *Continued*

Nursing Diagnosis	Expected Outcomes
III. *Potential for injury: infection and bleeding related to bone marrow depression*	B. Pt will experience minimal complications of bone marrow suppression as evidenced by return to normal temperature and neutrophil count and absence of major bleeding

Nursing Intervention

    f. Avoid invasive procedures, such as urinary catheterization, if possible

    g. Wash hands meticulously prior to entering room and between each physical contact with the pt; monitor that all other persons wash their hands prior to entering; ensure that the nurse caring for the pt does not care for any other pt who is infected

  2. Continually assess for presence of infection

    a. Monitor vital signs every 4 hours or more frequently if temperature is elevated

    b. Monitor absolute neutrophil count

    c. Inspect potential sites of infection: mouth, pharynx, rectum, wounds, intravenous sites, and others, remembering that usual signs of infection, such as pus and erythema, may be absent

    d. Monitor for changes in character, color, and amount of excretia (sputum, urine, stool)

    e. Report signs and symptoms of infection to physician and obtain cultures, administer antipyretics and antibiotics as ordered

  3. Instruct pt in stress-reducing activities to promote relaxation and satisfactory sleep/rest patterns

C. Institute platelet precautions for pt with platelet count less than 50,000/mm^3

  1. Protect pt from trauma and potential bleeding

    a. Place sign in nursing cardex that no IM or rectal medications should be administered, no aspirin or prostaglandin inhibiting medications should be administered, and no rectal temperatures should be taken

    b. Minimize number of venipunctures and apply pressure to site at least 5 minutes until bleeding stops

    c. Avoid invasive procedures, such as deep endotracheal suctioning, enemas, douches

    d. Teach pt to brush teeth with soft brush or sponge applicator to prevent trauma to gums; avoid flossing

    e. Provide safe environment, padding side rails when in use and removing clutter and obstructing furniture from room

    f. Prevent constipation by administering stool softeners as ordered, and encourage fluid intake of 3 liters per day

  2. Continually monitor for signs and symptoms of bleeding

    a. Minor bleeding, such as petechiae, ecchymoses, epistaxis; occult blood in stool, urine, emesis

    b. Major bleeding, such as hematemesis, melena, heavy vaginal bleeding; changes in orthostatic vital signs > 10 mmHg in blood pressure or increase in heart rate > 100 beats per minute; changes in neuro vital signs

Table 2 Standardized Nursing Care Plan for Patient
Experiencing Bone Marrow Depression *Continued*

Nursing Diagnosis	Expected Outcomes
IV. *Potential for altered tissue perfusion related to anemia*	IV. A. Pt will be without signs and symptoms of severe anemia
V. *Potential for constipation*	V. A. Pt will move bowels at least once every day
VI. *Potential for activity intolerance related to fatigue of anemia, malaise*	VI. A. Pt will maintain minimal activity

---

Nursing Intervention

    c. Monitor platelet count, hematocrit daily
    d. Notify MD re: signs and symptoms of bleeding, and transfuse platelets as ordered

---

IV. A. Assess signs and symptoms of anemia
    1. Hematocrit: mild (31–37%), moderate (25–30%), or severe (< 25%)
    2. Presence of symptoms of mild anemia (paleness, fatigue, slight dyspnea, palpitation, sweating on exertion); moderate anemia (increased severity of symptoms of mild anemia); and severe anemia (headache, dizziness, irritability, angina, dyspnea at rest, compensatory tachycardia, and tachypnea)
  B. Encourage pt to change positions gradually, slowly moving from lying to sitting position and sitting to standing position. Encourage slow, deep breathing during position changes
  C. Reassure pt that fatigue is related to anemia and hopefully will improve with transfusion
  D. Replace red blood cells as ordered, expecting that the 1 unit of RBCs will increase the hematocrit; washed or leukocyte-poor red blood cells are used to prevent antibody formation if the pt is planning to go for a bone marrow transplant
  E. Assess activity tolerance and need for oxygen for activity or at rest
  F. Review foods that are high in iron and folic acid and encourage pt to include these in the diet

---

V. A. Provide pt education about the goal and means of preventing constipation, such as stool softeners, oral fluids to 3 quarts per day, high-fiber diet, adequate exercise
  B. Discuss a bowel regime with physician to promote soft, regular bowel movements, especially if the pt is receiving narcotic analgesia

---

VI. A. Teach pt to increase rest and sleep periods and to alternate rest and activity periods
  B. Encourage pt to incorporate foods high in iron in diet, such as liver, eggs, lean meat, green leafy vegetables, carrots, and raisins
  C. Assess need for homemaker, home health aide, and visiting nurse at home
  D. Assess for psychological manifestations of fatigue:
    1. Depression
    2. Anxiety
    3. Loss of independence
    4. Decreased level of concentration
    5. Difficulty making decisions
  E. Teach pt to prioritize activities deciding what pt must do and those that can be delegated

Table 2 Standardized Nursing Care Plan for Patient
  Experiencing Bone Marrow Depression *Continued*

Nursing Diagnosis	Expected Outcomes
VI. *Potential for activity intolerance related to fatigue of anemia, malaise*	VI. A. Pt will maintain minimal activity

Nursing Intervention

    F. Teach pt to eat several small meals a day, and select high energy foods, such as potatoes, rice, pasta

    G. If pt able, teach pt to start and maintain an exercise program, starting slowly

        1. Gradually increase activity

        2. Low-impact exercises, such as stretching, muscle strengthening

        3. Cardiovascular exercises

Table 3 Standardized Nursing Care Plan for Patient
Experiencing Nausea and Vomiting

Nursing Diagnosis	Expected Outcomes
I. *Potential for altered nutrition, less than body requirements*	I. A. Pt will maintain weight within 5% of baseline B. Pt will be without nausea and vomiting and, if it occurs, it is minimal
II. *Potential for comfort alteration related to nausea and vomiting*	II. A. Pt will verbalize decreased anxiety and increased physical comfort

Nursing Intervention

I. A. Administer antiemetics prior to chemotherapy, and then regularly
       through expected duration of nausea and vomiting (depending on
       specific chemotherapeutic agent)
       1. Evaluate past effectiveness of antiemetic regime
       2. Evaluate need for continuing antiemetics 12–24 hrs after treatment
       3. Attempt to prevent nausea and vomiting during first treatment cycle
          to prevent anticipatory nausea and vomiting
    B. Administer chemotherapy at night or late afternoon if possible
    C. Experiment with eating patterns: suggest pt avoid eating prior to, during,
       and immediately after initial treatment to assess tolerance; discourage
       heavy, greasy, fatty, sweet, and spicy foods
    D. Encourage small, frequent, bland meals on day of therapy (if tolerates
       eating day of therapy) and increase fluid intake to 3 quarts/day
    E. Encourage pt to suck hard candy during therapy
    F. Provide environment that is clean, quiet, subdued, without odors
    G. Encourage weekly weighings; if pt unable to stabilize weight, refer to
       dietitian for intensive counseling, together with person responsible for
       doing the cooking
    H. Teach pt self-care measures
       1. Self-administration of antiemetics, including indications, dose,
          schedule, and potential side effects
       2. Dietary counseling encouraging bland, cool foods, cottage cheese,
          toast, if experiencing nausea and vomiting
       3. Encourage favorite high-calorie, high-protein, small, frequent feedings
          as tolerated; encourage fluids to 3 quarts/day, including chicken soup,
          Gatorade, sherbet, ginger ale
       4. Give pt copy of *Eating Hints* (NCI free publication), with ideas such as
          whole milk plus 1–2 T powdered milk in eggnogs, snacks to increase
          proteins, and calorie intake

II. A. Encourage pt to verbalize feelings re: prior treatments, if any, and
       significance of treatment to the pt
    B. Provide emotional support
    C. Consider anxiety-reducing drugs in antiemetic regime, such as lorazepam
    D. Minimize time pt is in waiting room or chemotherapy room
    E. Provide distraction using VCR/TV or radio as pt desires; for some pts,
       having a chaplain read the Psalms during therapy can be quite
       therapeutic
    F. Teach pt progressive muscle relaxation exercises and help pt to imagine
       peaceful past experiences; encourage fresh air
    G. Keep emesis basin within reach, provide cloth for face and hands if pt
       vomits

Table 3 Standardized Nursing Care Plan for Patient
Experiencing Nausea and Vomiting *Continued*

Nursing Diagnosis	Expected Outcomes
II. *Potential for comfort alteration related to nausea and vomiting* .	II. A. Pt will verbalize decreased anxiety and increased physical comfort
III. *Potential powerlessness*	III. A. Pt will have control over self-care activities
IV. *Potential for knowledge deficit of self-care measures*	IV. A. Pt will verbally repeat self-care measures and schedule for carrying them out
V. *Potential for injury related to nausea and vomiting (esophageal tears, bleeding)*	V. A. Pt will be free from injury B. Injury, if it occurs, will be detected early

Nursing Intervention
H. Assist pt with mouth care after emesis   I. Telephone pt, if treated as an output, the evening of or the day after chemotherapy administration to assess tolerance and comfort

III. A. Pt and family teaching re: potential side effects and self-care measures; offer pt and family *Chemotherapy and Use: A Self-Help Guide* (free NCI publication)
    B. Encourage pt to live as normal a lifestyle as possible, going out and engaging in usual activities; often doing something "nice" for oneself *after* treatment helps to minimize the distress and increase control
    C. Involve pt and family in appropriate decisions in treatment

IV. A. Instruct pt and family member in self-care measures
     1. Self-administration of antiemetics postchemotherapy
     2. Drink 3 quarts fluids per day, especially chicken soup, etc.
     3. Bland, cool, frequent, high-calorie, high-protein foods as tolerated
     4. Call health care provider for persistent nausea and vomiting
        > 3 times/day, inability to keep fluids down
    B. Use a positive approach in teaching re the potential side effect of nausea and vomiting, stressing efforts to prevent nausea and vomiting from occurring
    C. If nausea and vomiting occur, reassure pt that there are other antiemetic regimens that can be used to control, and hopefully prevent, it for the next cycle

V. A. Reinforce teaching pt to call clinic or health care provider if persistent nausea and vomiting occur, as well as if pain, bleeding, or any other abnormality occurs   B. If pt is taking steroids as part of chemotherapy or antiemetic regimen, teach pt to take pills with food

Table 4 Standardized Nursing Care Plan for Patient
              Experiencing Stomatitis

Nursing Diagnosis	Expected Outcomes
I. *Potential for altered oral mucous membranes*	I. A. Oral mucosa will remain pink, moist, intact, without debris
II. *Altered oral mucous membranes,* *Grade I* (generalized erythema) *Grade II* (small ulceration or white patches)	II. A. Oral mucosa will be pink, moist, intact, and painless within 5–7 days

Nursing Intervention

I.   A. Assess oral mucosa (baseline)
          1. Assess history of alcohol use, smoking
          2. Assess history of dental problems, oral hygiene practices, and prior or
              concurrent radiation to head or neck
          3. Perform oral exam
              a. Lips
              b. Upper inner lip and gums
              c. Tongue (dorsum, lateral borders, ventral surface)
              d. Inner cheeks (buccal mucosa)
              e. Hard and soft palate
              f. Floor of mouth
              g. Oral pharynx
          4. Assess amount, consistency of saliva
          5. Assess condition of teeth
      B. Assess nutritional status
      C. Initiate and discuss dental referral as needed prior to therapy
      D. Instruct in oral hygiene self-care measures (see IV. Potential for
          knowledge deficit)

II.   A. Assess oral mucosa q shift or at each clinic visit; document size and
          location of abnormality and intervention
      B. Assess comfort and ability to eat, drink
      C. Institute oral hygiene q 2 hrs during day and q 6 hrs during night
          1. Warm normal saline rinses *unless* crusts, debris, thick mucus or saliva;
              then use sodium bicarbonate (1 tsp in 8 oz water) q 4 hrs alternating
              with warm saline rinses q 4 hrs
          2. (Warm) sterile normal saline rinses if WBC $< 1000/mm^3$
          3. Reserve hydrogen peroxide (1:4 strength) for *resistant,* thick secretions
              or white patches (*candida*) and resistant debris, and rinse afterward
              with water
      D. Encourage flossing qd and brushing with soft-bristled brush pc and hs
          unless plt $< 40,000/mm^3$ or WBC $< 1500/mm^3$
      E. Encourage pt to remove dentures during oral hygiene rinsing and if
          irritating mucosa
      F. Encourage pt to moisten lips with medicated lip ointment, water-soluble
          lubricating jelly, or lanolin
      G. Encourage pt to avoid citrus fruits and juices, spicy foods, hot foods, and
          to eat bland, cool foods
      H. Discuss use of antifungal therapy if candidiasis present

Table 4 Standardized Nursing Care Plan for Patient
Experiencing Stomatitis *Continued*

Nursing Diagnosis	Expected Outcomes
III. *Altered oral mucous membranes, Grade III* (confluent ulcerations with white patches > 25% or unable to drink liquids) *Grade IV* (hemorrhagic ulcerations and/or unable to drink liquids and eat solid food)	III. A. Oral mucosa will heal within 10–14 days, and white patches (*candida*) are absent
IV. *Potential for knowledge deficit, re: risk for stomatitis and self-care management*	IV. A. Pt verbally repeats steps of self-assessment B. Pt demonstrates self-care techniques (mouth rinse, brushing, flossing)
V. *Pain related to stomatitis*	V. A. Pt states relief from oral pain

Nursing Intervention

III. A. Assess oral mucosa q 4 hrs for evidence of infection, response to therapy
      B. Assess ability to eat, drink, communicate
      C. Assess level of comfort, discomfort
      D. Culture ulcerated areas that appear infected
      E. Cleanse mouth q 2 hrs while awake, q 4 hrs during night
          1. Alternate warm saline mouth rinse with antifungal or antibacterial oral suspension q 2 hrs
          2. Use sodium bicarbonate solution for thick secretions, debris; if ineffective in removing debris, use 1:4 hydrogen peroxide followed by water or saline rinse
      F. Suggest soft sponge-tipped applicator to cleanse teeth, mouth pc and hs
      G. Apply lip lubricant q 2 hrs

IV.   A. Instruct pt in stomatitis as potential side effect of chemotherapy as appropriate
      B. Instruct pt in daily oral exam
          1. Use of mirror and self-exam
          2. Signs and symptoms to report (burning, redness, blisters, ulcers; difficulty swallowing; swelling of lips, tongue; pain)
      C. Instruct pt in oral care
          1. Remove dentures; wash and rinse mouth; and then replace
          2. Floss daily with unwaxed dental floss
          3. Brush with soft toothbrush and nonabrasive toothpaste pc and hs
          4. Rinse with water, saline, dilute sodium bicarbonate solution, or mouthwash without alcohol
          5. Avoid oral irritants (tobacco, alcohol, poorly fitting dentures, mouthwashes containing alcohol)
      D. Instruct pt in self-care q 2 hrs if actual stomatitis occurs
          1. Cleansing solution of warm normal saline or sodium bicarbonate solution unless resistant thick secretions, debris; then can use 1:4 hydrogen peroxide with water rinse following
          2. Medication application as indicated
          3. High-calorie, high-protein, cool, bland foods
          4. Small, frequent feedings; fluids to 3 L/day

V.   A. Use mild analgesic q 2 hrs, timing 15 mins ac; gargles must be swished 2 min
          1. Viscous zylocaine 2% gargles, 10–15 cc swish/spit q 3 hrs, duration 20 mins (max 120 mg/24 hrs)
          2. Orabase emollient for local relief
          3. 1:1:1 viscous zylocaine:diphenhydramine HCl (12.5 mg/ml): Kaopectate swish and swallow q 2–4 hrs

Table 4 Standardized Nursing Care Plan for Patient
Experiencing Stomatitis *Continued*

Nursing Diagnosis	Expected Outcomes
V. *Pain related to stomatitis*	V. A. Pt states relief from oral pain
VI. *Impaired verbal communication related to pain, increased or thickened saliva*	VI. A. Pt will communicate needs effectively
VII. *Potential for altered nutrition: less than body requirements related to pain of mucositis*	VII. A. Pt will regain baseline weight within 5%
VIII. *Potential for infection*	VIII. A. Pt will be free of infection B. Infection will be detected early and treated
IX. *Potential for altered tissue perfusion related to hemorrhage*	IX. A. Pt will be without oral bleeding B. Bleeding will be detected early and terminated

Nursing Intervention

      4. Benzocaine 20%—apply directly or swish and spit (duration 20 mins)
      5. Dyclonine HCl (Dyclone) 0.5% 15 mins ac: 5–10 cc swish for
         2 mins, gargle and spit, onset 10 mins, duration 1 hr
  B. Parenteral analgesics may be necessary, including morphine infusion

VI. A. Assess pt's ability to communicate
     B. If secretion is thick, copious, instruct pt in tonsil-tip suctioning technique
     C. Develop satisfactory communication tool if pt unable to talk (i.e., magic slate, writing message)
     D. Respond promptly to pt call light

VII. A. Premedicate with analgesics 15 mins ac
     B. Encourage high-calorie, high-protein, small, frequent feedings with cool, bland liquid or pureed foods; also, creative popsicles, custards
     C. If inability to eat persists, discuss with MD need for enteral, parenteral nutrition
     D. Encourage popsicles, ice creams as desired
     E. Discourage citrus juices, fruits, hot and spicy foods, rough or hard foods

VIII. A. Assess oral mucosa q 4–8 hrs for s/s infection—culture any suspicious sites
      B. Monitor vs, T q 4 hrs; if outpatient, teach pt to monitor temperature at least BID
      C. Encourage pt to cleanse oral mucosa prior to administration of antibiotic or antifungal medication—keep NPO for 15–30 mins p medication administration
      D. Consider administration of antifungal or antibiotic as frozen popsicle if extreme pain, as this can decrease discomfort
      E. Administer systemic antibiotics if ordered

IX. A. Assess for s/s bleeding in gingiva, mucosa
    B. Remove dentures, partial plates
    C. If *bleeding*, monitor platelet count, hematocrit
      1. Transfuse platelets as ordered
      2. Topical thrombin, aminocaproic acid, or microfibrillar collagen may be ordered (Peterson 1984)
      3. Leave clots undisturbed—discontinue mechanical oral care
    D. Use sponge-tipped applicator rather than toothbrush if platelets $< 50,000/mm^3$ to minimize trauma to gingiva, mucosa
    E. Encourage liquid, cool or cold, high-calorie, high-protein supplements as tolerated; pt should be NPO if bleeding

Table 4 Standardized Nursing Care Plan for Patient
             Experiencing Stomatitis *Continued*

Nursing Diagnosis	Expected Outcomes
X. *Xerostomia* (uncommon)	X. A. Pt will have moist mucosa with thin secretions

Nursing Intervention

X.   A. Encourage frequent mouth moisturizing with ice chips, artificial saliva
        (containing carboxymethyl cellulose)
     B. Oral hygiene pc and hs
     C. Encourage fluids as tolerated, offer fluids every 1–2 hrs
     D. Discourage mucosal irritants (smoking, alcohol)
     E. Encourage soft, moist foods with sauces
     F. Encourage use of sugarless candy or gum to stimulate saliva production
     G. Increase air moisture as needed by humidifier or vaporizer
     H. Oral assessment q day, as xerostomia may precede stomatitis (erythema)

Table 5 Standardized Nursing Care Plan for Patient Experiencing Diarrhea

Nursing Diagnosis		Expected Outcomes	
I.	*Potential for altered nutrition: less than body requirements*	I.	A. Pt will maintain baseline weight within 5% B. Serum electrolytes will be within normal limits
II.	*Potential for fluid volume deficit*	II.	A. Pt's skin will have normal turgor B. Mucous membranes will be moist
III.	*Diarrhea* A. Mild/moderate (4–6 stools/day) B. Severe (> 6 stools/day)	III.	A. Pt will have < 4 stools/day
IV.	*Potential for impaired mucosal and skin integrity, perianal skin, related to diarrhea*	IV.	A. Skin and perianal mucosa will remain intact
V.	*Potential for pain*	V.	A. Pt will verbalize decreased pain

Nursing Intervention

I. A. Assess pt's usual weight, dietary preferences, and usual pattern of bowel elimination
    B. Monitor intake/output, daily weight, calorie count as appropriate
    C. Encourage high-calorie, high-protein, low-residue diet in small, frequent meals (cottage cheese, cream cheese, yogurt, broth, fish, poultry, custard, cooked cereals, peeled apples, macaroni, cooked vegetables)
    D. If diarrhea is severe, recommend liquid diet
    E. Discourage foods that stimulate peristalsis (bran, whole-grain bread, fried food, fruit juices, raw vegetables, nuts, rich pastry, caffeine-containing foods and drinks)
    F. Encourage foods high in potassium as appropriate (bananas, baked potatoes, asparagus tips); monitor serum potassium, other electrolytes

II. A. Encourage 3 liters of fluid/day, especially bouillon, Gatorade
    B. If nutritional supplements are needed, recommend lactose-free or low-osmolality products
    C. Monitor intake/output

III. A. Assess bowel sounds and abdomen for rigidity
    B. Assess frequency, consistency, and volume of stooling and document. Have pt maintain diary if an outpatient
    C. Administer antidiarrheal medication as ordered; assess response to therapy; assess need for antispasmodics, antianxiety (anxiolytic) medications
    D. Instruct pt in self-care measures
      1. Self-administration of medications
      2. Low-residue diet, fluids to 3 L/day
      3. Perianal skin care
      4. Alternate rest/activity periods
    E. Discuss interruption of chemotherapy with physician

IV. A. Assess perineal, perianal skin, and mucous membranes for integrity and for s/s irritation
    B. Recommend sitz baths p̄ each stool, if diarrhea severe
    C. Provide skin cleansing with water and mild soap p̄ each stool, and application of skin barrier as needed, if pt unable to perform care; otherwise instruct pt in self-care
    D. Apply topical anesthetic as needed
    E. Use absorbent pads under pt to prevent maceration of skin

V. A. Give symptomatic treatment to minimize or alleviate pain

Table 5 Standardized Nursing Care Plan for Patient
Experiencing Diarrhea *Continued*

Nursing Diagnosis	Expected Outcomes
VI. *Potential for fatigue*	VI. A. Pt will verbalize decreased fatigue
VII. *Potential for activity intolerance*	VII. A. Pt will participate in activities important to him or her

Nursing Intervention
VI.   A. Assess energy level and help pt to plan activities when energy level is maximal
B. Assess for changes in lifestyle necessitated by diarrhea
C. Encourage pt to alternate rest and activity periods
D. Provide care that pt is unable to perform; encourage pt to involve family if pt is at home; consider/refer community agencies as needed (for homemaker, home health aide) if diarrhea is severe and resistant to treatment
E. Assist pt in determining activity priorities and measures to conserve energy
VII.   A. Activities will be consistent with pt's level of well-being

Table 6 Potential Hepatotoxicity of Chemotherapeutic Agents

Drug	Toxicity
amsacrine (investigational)	Mild increase in bilirubin in 20–40% patients; rare hepatic failure
Nitrosoureas (carmustine, lomustine)	Increased LFTs, normalize in 1 wk Rare veno-occlusive disease in BMT
streptozocin	Increased LFTs (in ~ 15% patients)
Antimetabolites methotrexate	Increased SGOT, LDH (short, frequent doses or high doses); fibrosis, cirrhosis (long-term use)
6-mercaptopurine	Increased bilirubin, SGOT, alkaline phosphatase; cholestasis, necrosis
cytosine arabinoside	Increased LFTs
hydroxyurea	Rare increase in LFTs, hepatitis
capecitabine	Increase in bilirubin, alkaline phosphatase
Antibiotics mithramycin	Acute necrosis, altered LFTs, clotting factors
Bisantrene	Rare hepatitis
Enzymes L-asparaginase	Fatty changes, with decreased albumin, clotting factor synthesis; impaired handling of lipids
Miscellaneous dacarbazine	Transient increase in SGPT, SGOT, bilirubin (diffuse hepatocellular dysfunction); also reported veno-occlusive disease—rare
Alkylating agents chlorambucil	Hepatitis, dysfunction
cisplatin	Steatosis and cholestasis
busulfan	Cholestatic jaundice
Plant alkaloids paclitaxel	Usually mild increase in LFTs
doxetaxel	Increased bilirubin and alkaline phosphatase

Sources: Perry, M. C. (1984). Hepatotoxicity. In M.C. Perry and J.W. Yarbro (Eds.): *Toxicity of Chemotherapy.* Orlando,FL: Grune and Stratton, 297–312; Dorr, R.T., and Fritz, W.L. (1981). *Cancer Chemotherapy Handbook*, New York: Elsevier, 130–133; Goodman, M.S. (1987). *Cancer: Chemotherapy and Care*, Evansville, IN: Bristol-Myers USP&NG, 32–33.

Comments

Appears dose related; hold drug for prolonged elevations
Occurs with usual and high doses; does not usually require treatment

Resolve within 1 mo after treatment stops; avoid use in patients with Laennec's
    cirrhosis or preexisting liver disease
Usually not given to patients with preexisting liver disease; discontinue drug if
    increased LFTs occur—usually related to doses > 2 mg/kg/day
Dose reduce for hyperbilirubinemia

Stop drug or reduce dose

Usually improves after treatment stopped, resolving over days to weeks

Treatment not usually necessary

Stop drug

Incidence 7–22%; dose reduce if severe toxicity
Stop drug if severe toxicity

Table 7 Relative Risks of Chemotherapeutic Agents:
Nephrotoxicity

Drug	Pathophysiology
I. *High risk of immediate nephrotoxicity*	
A. cisplatin	A. Proximal and distal renal tubule injury produces tubular necrosis, focal degeneration of basement membrane, hyaline droplet deposits in renal tubules 1. *Mild,* reversible with low doses 2. *Severe,* permanent damage with high doses and multiple courses
B. High-dose methotrexate	B. Drug crystallizes or precipitates in renal tubules and collecting ducts; directly affects renal tubular cells; directly affects afferent vascular supply, resulting in $\downarrow$ glomerular filtration rate (GFR) 1. Rare and reversible with short-term low doses 2. Occasional long-term, low-dose permanent dysfunction 3. High incidence with high dose, usually reversible but with significant systemic drug toxicity
C. streptozocin	C. 10–20% of intact, active drug is excreted by kidneys, with primary injury on renal tubules and glomeruli, resulting in tubular interstitial nephritis and tubular atrophy 1. Low doses produce transient, reversible damage 2. Continued therapy can lead to severe and permanent chronic renal failure 3. Dose-limiting factor
D. High-dose mithramycin	D. Direct damage to renal tubules, causing distal and proximal tubule necrosis 1. Rare with low dose 2. High incidence with high dose and may be permanent
E. ifosfamide	E. Renal toxicity incidence $\sim 6\%$, apparently related to tubular damage 1. Laboratory abnormalities usually transient

Laboratory Abnormalities	Nursing Interventions
A. ↑ BUN and creatinine, ↓creatinine clearance, azotemia, ↓ serum magnesium, ↓ serum calcium; renal wasting with hypermagnesuria, hypercalcuria, proteinuria, enzymuria	A. 1. Saline hydration at least 100–150 ml/hr 2. Diuresis with mannitol or furosemide 3. Post-treatment hydration of at least 3 L/day 4. Prevent dehydration and vomiting

B. ↑ BUN and creatinine, oliguria/anuria, azotemia, acidosis, hypokalemia, anemia, osteomalacia, hypophosphatemia, aminoaciduria	B. 1. Vigorous hydration to maintain high urine flow
	2. Alkalinize urine to pH ≥ 7.0
	3. Prevent dehydration, vomiting
	4. Prevent systemic drug toxicity
	   a. Leucovorin rescue *exactly* on time until methotrexate level < 5 × 10^{-8}M
	   b. Effusions should be drained *prior* to drug administration
	5. Eliminate concomitant administration of sulfonamides, salicylates, probenecid

C. ↑ BUN and creatinine, ↓ creatinine clearance, hypophosphatemia, hypokalemia, hyperchloremia, proteinuria, glycosuria, aminoaciduria, phosphaturia	C. 1. Adequate hydration during and 24 hrs after treatment 2. Prevent vomiting, dehydration 3. Assess 24-hr urine creatinine clearance before treatment
D. ↑ BUN and serum creatinine, azotemia, proteinuria, hypophosphatemia, hypomagnesemia, hypokalemia, hypocalcemia	D. 1. Monitor renal function 2. No prevention strategies; however, high doses rarely administered
E. ↑ BUN and serum creatinine, ↓ urine creatinine clearance, rare proteinuria, acidosis 1. Microscopic hematuria	E. 1. Monitor kidney function (laboratory tests), vigorous hydration 2. Uroprotector must be administered with ifosfamide (i.e., mesna)

Table 7 Relative Risks of Chemotherapeutic Agents:
Nephrotoxicity *Continued*

Drug	Pathophysiology
	2. Bladder irritation, consisting of hemorrhagic cystitis, dysuria, and urinary frequency, occurs in 6–92% of patients without uroprotection 3. Urotoxicity is dose dependent
II. *High risk of nephrotoxicity from long-term use* A. nitrosoureas (BCNU, CCNU, MeCCNU)	A. Postulated that drug binds irreversibly to amino acid residues → glomerular and tubular damage, decrease in kidney size 1. Uncommon with doses < 1000 mg/m^2 2. In high dose, chronic renal failure may occur
B. mitomycin C	B. Postulated drug interferes with DNA synthesis and induces immune complex deposits, damaging glomeruli and tubules 1. Cumulative toxicity 2. Mild and reversible to fatal renal failure (i.e., if hemolytic uremic syndrome [HUS] develops) 3. Renal vasculitis may be increased with concurrent 5-fluorouracil administration
III. *Moderate risk of nephrotoxicity* A. cyclophosphamide	A. 1. Drug metabolites may injure collecting ducts and distal renal tubules, causing impaired water excretion and dilutional hyponatremia (SIADH) at high doses (> 50 mg/kg) 2. Drug metabolites irritate stretched bladder capillaries, causing hemorrhagic cystitis

Laboratory Abnormalities	Nursing Interventions
	a. Assess urine for presence of RBC prior to subsequent dosing b. Manufacturer recommends urinalysis be assessed prior to each drug dose 1) If microscopic hematuria present (> 10 RBC/high power field), dose should be held until complete resolution 2) Further drug administration should be given with vigorous oral/parenteral hydration
A. ↑ BUN and serum creatinine, ↓ glomerular filtration rate (GFR), azotemia, proteinuria	A. 1. No prevention strategies; suggest hydration during and after drug administration (oral fluids to 3 L/day for 24 hrs) 2. Frequent long-term follow-up, as renal failure may occur up to 5 years later
B. 1. ↑ BUN, azotemia, proteinuria 2. HUS: hypertension, hematuria, anemia, thrombocytopenia	B. 1. No prevention strategies 2. Suggest hydration during and 24 hrs post-treatment 3. Assess renal function
A. SIADH: Lab values of water intoxication: serum hyponatremia, ↑ urine osmolality ↓ serum osmolality, ↓ urinary output	A. 1. Monitor electrolytes, treat SIADH if it occurs 2. Prevent by aggressive hydration (at least 3 L/day) 3. Encourage pt to void at least q 2–3 hrs 4. Do not administer at noc

Table 7 Relative Risks of Chemotherapeutic Agents: Nephrotoxicity *Continued*

Drug	Pathophysiology
	3. Preventable
	4. Dose-limiting
B. Low-dose methotrexate	B. See pathophysiology—high-dose methotrexate
C. 5-azacytidine investigational	C. Tubular damage and renal insufficiency possible when given in combination with other drugs
D. High-dose 6-thioguanine	D. High dose (oral or IV) appears to induce reversible toxicity, possibly by inhibiting purine metabolism
E. L-asparaginase	E. Prerenal azotemia

IV. *Low-risk of nephrotoxicity*

    A. Anthracyclines (doxorubicin in high doses, daunorubicin)

    B. Low-dose mithramycin

    C. Tenoposide (VM-26)

    D. 5-fluorouracil

    E. vincristine (SIADH, ↑ serum Na^{++}, inappropriate urinary sodium wasting)

    F. 6-mercaptopurine (hematuria, requires dose reduction)

    G. carboplatin (rare tubular damage)

    H. hydroxyurea (mild, reversible, requires dosage reduction)

Source: Modified from Lydon, J. (1986). Nephrotoxicity of cancer treatment, *Oncology Nursing Forum, 13*(2): 68–77.

Laboratory Abnormalities	Nursing Interventions
B. Hemorrhagic cystitis: urinary frequency, urgency, dysuria, hematuria	B. No nursing interventions
C. ↑ BUN and creatinine, azotemia, acidosis, hyperphosphatemia, hypomagnesemia, hypocalcemia, glycosuria, sodium wasting, aminoaciduria	C. No prevention strategies known; assess renal function prior to each dose
D. ↑ BUN and creatinine, azotemia	D. No prevention strategies; monitor renal function studies prior to each dose
E. ↑ BUN	E. Use cautiously with nephrotoxic antibiotics; monitor renal function studies

Table 8 Standardized Nursing Care Plan for Patient Experiencing Alopecia

Nursing Diagnosis	Defining Characteristics
I. *Potential body image disturbances related to alopecia*	I. A. Chemotherapy agents attack rapidly dividing normal as well as abnormal cells. The cells and tissues responsible for hair growth have a high mitotic rate and are sensitive to the effects of chemotherapy. The potential depends on the activity of the drug in specific phases of replication. The drugs most commonly implicated in causing alopecia because they affect the S phase of the cell cycle are

bleomycin   ifosfamide
cisplatin   melphalan
cyclophosphamide   methotrexate
dactinomycin   mitomycin-C
daunorubicin   paclitaxel
docetaxel   topotecan
doxorubicin   vinbastine
etoposide   vincristine
5-fluorouracil   vinorelbine
hydroxyurea

B. Doxorubicin causes alopecia in greater than 80% of pts treated, usually within 21 days. Alopecia caused from cyclophosphamide depends on dose (occurs more frequently with higher doses). Alopecia from methotrexate is also dose related. With 5-fluorouracil, thinning of eyebrows and loss of eyebrows may be observed in addition to loss of scalp hair. Range of alopecia may be from thinning of hair to a total body hair loss.

C. Regrowth depends on schedule of treatments and doses administered. Usually regrowth begins 2–3 months after cessation of therapy.

D. Whole-brain radiation (5000–7000 rads) usually results in permanent alopecia as a result of permanent damage to hair follicles Radiation to lower levels of brain may not cause permanent alopecia.

Expected Outcomes	**Nursing Intervention**

I. A. Pt, significant other, or family member will verbalize an understanding of factors that cause alopecia (chemotherapy, radiation therapy)
 	
B. Pt will discuss the impact of alopecia on his or her lifestyle
 	
C. Pt will demonstrate knowledge of appropriate measures to minimize alopecia
	I. A. Assess pt for being at risk for developing alopecia
	B. Instruct pt about hair loss, temporary or permanent, and the effects of chemotherapy on hair follicles
	C. Instruct pt on the potential for regrowth and for the potential change in color and texture
	D. Assess the impact of alopecia on pt
	E. Encourage verbalization of feelings
	F. Encourage pt to cut long hair short so as to minimize the shock of alopecia
	G. Discuss various measures to take during hair loss: wigs, scarves, hats, turban, use of makeup to highlight other features, baseball caps, cowboy hats
	H. Encourage support groups with people experiencing alopecia
	I. Encourage pt to help maintain personal identity by wearing own clothes in hospital and retaining social contacts
	J. Instruct pt on proper scalp care
	  1. Use baby shampoo or mild soap
	  2. Use soft brush to minimize pulling at hair
	  3. Use mineral oil or Vitamin A&D ointment to reduce itching
	  4. Always use a sunscreen when exposed to sun (SPF 15 or higher)
	K. If pt loses eyelashes or eyebrows instruct pt to use methods for protecting eyes (eyeglasses, hats with wide brim)

Table 9 Standardized Nursing Care Plan for Patient Experiencing Sexual Dysfunction

Nursing Diagnosis	Defining Characteristics

I. *Sexual dysfunction related to disease process, treatment, or infertility*	I. A. Cancer pts often experience some sexual alteration as a result of physical or psychological insults by the disease process, diagnosis, side effects of chemotherapy, surgical intervention, or radiation
	B. Some chemotherapy causes sexual infertility:
	    chlorambucil
	    cyclophosphamide
	    doxorubicin
	    cytarabine
	    procarbazine
	    vinblastine
	C. Dimensions altered by cancer therapy may affect behavior used to express sexual identity

Expected Outcomes	Nursing Intervention

I. A. Pt will demonstrate knowledge of factors that may potentially affect sexuality
B. Pt will verbalize the potential impact of diagnosis on sexual activity
C. Pt will maintain satisfying sex role and sexual self-image
D. Pt will identify strategies used to minimize sexual dysfunction
E. Pt or significant other will identify other measures used for sexual expression
	I. A. Establish a trusting relationship with the pt
	B. Assess pt's knowledge regarding the effects of the disease and treatment on sexuality
	C. Provide a comfortable, relaxed environment in which to discuss with pt the effects of disease and treatment on sexuality
	D. Allow pt and significant other to verbalize perceptions of how disease and treatment will affect sexual function and sexuality
	E. Discuss strategies to minimize sexual dysfunction
	  1. Alternative forms of sexual expression
	  2. Alternative positions to decrease pain and prevent injury
	  3. Encourage sexual activity when energy levels are highest (in morning, after naps)
	  4. Help pt to recognize sexual feelings and urges
	  5. Include sexual partner in counseling and teaching
	  6. Explain effects of drugs and treatment on fertility
	  7. Refer for further counseling, if necessary
	F. Discuss options regarding alternative methods of family planning
	  1. Foster parenthood
	  2. Adoption
	  3. Provide information on sperm banking

Table 10 Drugs That Can Induce Pulmonary Toxicity

Drug	Risk Factors
Incidence: Frequent	
bleomycin	Age > 70 Dose: At 400–500 U constant low rate, at 500 U rate increases but can occur at low doses High O_2 exposure, thoracic radiation, and renal dysfunction
carmustine (BCNU)	Preexisting lung disease, tobacco use, industrial exposure, possible synergism with cyclophosphamide and thoracic radiation Dose: > 1000 mg/m², linear toxicity effect
Incidence: Moderate	
busulfan	Thoracic radiation: 500 mg may be threshold dose for toxicity
methotrexate delayed	Daily and weekly schedules most likely to result in toxicity
Incidence: Moderate to low	
cyclophosphamide	None identified, but frequently reported in patients with Hodgkin's and non-Hodgkin's lymphoma; possibly related to concurrent bleomycin
mitomycin	High concentration of O_2
fludarabine	Concurrent administration with pentostatin (deoxycofomycin) has resulted in fatal pulmonary toxicity
Incidence: Low	
chlorambucil	None identified, duration of therapy 6 mos to > 2 yrs; total dose > 2 gm
cytosine arabinoside	None identified
melphalan	None identified, total dose 80 mg to > 3 gm; duration of therapy 2–83 mos

Signs and Symptoms/Comments

Dry cough, dyspnea, tachypnea, fever, and rales, which can progress to coarse rhonchi and occasional pleural friction rub

Incidence: 5–11%

Variable, none to dyspnea; dry cough; bibasilar crepitant rales
Incidence: 20–30%
Mortality: 24–80%

Insidious onset; dyspnea, dry cough, and fever progressive over weeks to months; bilateral basilar crepitant rales and tachypnea
Prodromal symptoms; headache and malaise, dyspnea, dry cough, and fever for days to weeks; tachypnea, cyanosis, rales, skin eruptions—16%; eosinophilia—50%; steroid therapy may be helpful

Dyspnea, fever, dry cough, tachypnea, scattered rales, rarely chest pain or pleural rub

Progressive dyspnea, nonproductive cough, bibasilar rales; may occur with low doses and after first dose; may be associated with renal toxicity
Pneumonia occurs in 16–22% of patients. Pulmonary hypersensitivity is characterized by dyspnea, cough, interstitial pulmonary infiltrate

Dyspnea, dry cough, fever developing over 1–2 mos, bibasilar rales, anorexia, fatigue
Dyspnea and tachypnea develop during or after therapy, associated with GI lesions; rare pulmonary edema
Rapid progressive dyspnea and fever over 2–10 days; tachypnea, rales common

Table 10 Drugs That Can Induce Pulmonary Toxicity *Continued*

Drug	Risk Factors
Incidence: Rare	
Chlorozotocin	None identified
etoposide	Questionable synergism with methotrexate
lomustine	Dose: > 1100 mg/m^2 Questionable synergism with other pulmonary-toxic chemotherapy
mercaptopurine methotrexate	None identified
procarbazine	None identified: potential risk for hypersensitivity-prone individuals
semustine	None identified
Spirogermanium	None identified: potential risk for patients previously treated with other chemotherapy or thoracic radiation
teniposide	Previous treatment with XRT to spinal axis and BCNU
vindesine and vinblastine	Seen in patients treated simultaneously with mitomycin
Zinostatin	None identified

Source: Modified from Wickham, R. (1986). Pulmonary toxicity secondary to cancer treatment, *Oncology Nursing Forum, 13*(5): 69–76.

Signs and Symptoms/Comments

Exertional dyspnea, rales, fatigue
Fever, dyspnea, cough, dry rales, cyanosis, tachypnea
Dyspnea, tachypnea, weight loss, anorexia

Acute respiratory distress
Pulmonary edema, acute onset of dyspnea, tachypnea 6–12 hrs after oral or
    intrathecal (IT) drug administration
Fever, chills, eosinophilia, rash, cough, dyspnea, progressive pulmonary
    insufficiency; rapid recovery after discontinuation of drug
Exertional dyspnea, rales, pleural friction rub
Progressive cough, dyspnea, fatigue, and fever; onset of symptoms insidious

Dyspnea, cyanosis, tachypnea
Acute onset; dyspnea and cough, tachypnea, rales

Dry cough, hemoptysis, progressive pulmonary insufficiency

Table 11 Chemotherapeutic Agents Associated with Cardiac Toxicities

Drug	Dosage	Cardiac Toxicity
aminoglutethimide	250 mg po qid	Hypotension, tachycardia
amsacrine (AMSA)	100 mg/m^2 IV qd × 3 or 75–150 mg/m^2 IV qd × 5	Ventricular fibrillation Cardiomyopathy
cisplatin	Unknown	Cardiac ischemia
cisplatin-based combination therapy	Unknown	Arterial occlusion events, MI, CVA
cyclophosphamide	120–270 mg/kg × 1–4 days	Hemorrhagic myocardial necrosis
dactinomycin	0.25 mg/m^2 × 5 days	Cardiomyopathy
daunorubicin	400–500 mg/m^2 (lifetime dose)	Transient EKG changes Cardiomyopathy
diethylstilbestrol (DES)	5 mg q d	Thromboembolic myocardial infarction
doxorubicin	450–550 mg/m^2 (lifetime dose)	Transient EKG changes Cardiomyopathy
doxydoxorubicin (DXDX; synthetic anthracycline)	25–30 mg/m^2	CHF (cumulative dose-related cardiotoxicity with 250 mg/m^2)
4'-epidoxorubicin (anthracycline analogue)	100mg/m^2 q 3 wks or 60 mg/m^2 dL, 8 q 28 days; 900mg/m^2 (lifetime dose)	Transient EKG changes, ventricular extrasystole CHF
estramustine	600 mg/m^2 po in 3 divided doses	Hypertension, angina, myocardial infarction, arrhythmias, pulmonary emboli
estrogens	5 mg qd	CHF with ischemic heart disease, thromboembolic CVA

Occurence	Comments
10%	Can occur at any time during treatment.
5%	Risk is increased by accumulative dose of greater than 900 mg/m^2 or greater than 200 mg/m^2 of AMSA in 48 hrs. Increased incidence with previous anthracycline exposure. Cardiac toxicity is enhanced by preexisting hypokalemia.
Rare	
Rare	Reports of myocardial infarction (MI), cerebrovascular accident (CVA) after treatment with cisplatin, velban, bleomycin, etoposide.
Rare	Occurs with induced myelosuppression for bone marrow transplantation. Potentiates anthracycline-induced cardiomyopathy.
Rare	Seen with previous anthracycline exposure.
0–41% 1.5%	Increased risk with concomitant cyclophosphamide or previous chest irradiation. Young children and the elderly are most susceptible.
CVA, frequent	Risk decreased by decreasing dose to 1 mg qd.
2.2% 1–5%	Same as for daunorubicin.
Rare	Radionuclide ejected fraction performed after pt receives 150 mg/m^2 cumulative dose. Repeat at each dose of 250 mg/m^2.
1%	Spectrum of activity is similar to doxorubicin. Incidence of CHF is 1.6% when cumulative when doses of 700 mg/m^2 are given.
10–15%	Increased risk with history of cardiovascular disease.
39%	Increased risk with history of cardiovascular disease.

Table 11 Chemotherapeutic Agents Associated with Cardiac Toxicities *Continued*

Drug	Dosage	Cardiac Toxicity
etoposide (VP-16)	Unknown	Myocardial infarction
fluorouracil	12–15 mg/kg q wk; 1000 mg/m^2 qd 1–4 days as continuous infusion	Angina 3–18 hrs after drug administered; or during high-dose continuous infusion
mithramycin	25–50 mg/kg IV qod × 3–8 days	Cardiomyopathy
mitomycin	15 mg/m^2 q 6–8 wks	Cardiomyopathy
mitoxantrone	a. 12–14 mg/m^2 q 3 wks b. 100 mg/m^2 lifetime dose with prior exposure to anthracyclines c. 160 mg/m^2 lifetime dose without prior exposure to anthracyclines	a. Transient EKG changes b. Decreased ejection fraction c. CHF
paclitaxel	135 mg/m^2 or higher	Asymptomatic bradycardia; rarely may progress to heart block Rarely, chest pain, brief ventricular tachycardia or supraventricular tachycardia
vincristine and vinblastine	Unknown	Myocardial infarction

Source: Adapted with permission from Kaszyk, L. K. (1986). Cardiac toxicity associated with cancer therapy, *Oncology Nursing Forum, 13*(4): 81–88.

Occurence	Comments
Rare	May be worsened with prior mediastinal XRT and preexisting coronary artery disease.
Rare	Not necessarily with preexisting cardiovascular disease. Can recur with subsequent doses. Cardiac enzymes are normal.
Rare	Exacerbates subclinical anthracycline-induced cardiotoxicity.
Rare	Increased risk with previous chest irradiation or anthracycline exposure. Synergistic with anthracyclines.
a. 28% b. 44% c. 2.1–12.5%	Increased risk of cardiomyopathy with previous anthracycline exposure, chest irradiation, or cardiovascular disease. CHF has occurred in pts who have not received prior anthracycline therapy.
29%	Asymptomatic bradycardia may occur during or up to 8 hrs after paclitaxel infusion; one fatal myocardial infarction has been reported.
Rare	Phenomena not well described.

Table 12 Standardized Nursing Care Plan for the
          Patient Experiencing Neuropathy

Nursing Diagnosis	Expected Outcome
I. *Potential for injury related to ↓ sensitivity to temperature, gait disturbance, ↓ proprioception*	I. A. Pt will be without injury B. Pt will report changes in tactile and proprioceptive function C. Pt will develop safe measures to compensate for losses
II. *Potential for impaired self-care related to tactile and proprioception dysfunction*	II. A. Pt will identify activities of self-care that are difficult B. Pt will identify strategies to meet needs
III. *Potential for alteration in comfort related to painful paresthesias*	III. A. Pt will have decreased pain

Nursing Intervention

I. A. Assess integrity of *tactile* and *proprioceptive* functions
      1. Sensory perception to light touch, pinprick, vibration, temperature; vision, color vision
      2. Pt's ability to tolerate light touch, cool water, presence of numbness and tingling, presence of painful sensations
      3. Proprioception testing of station, gait, deep tendon reflexes, muscle weakness or atrophy, and balance
      4. Pt's ability to sense placement of body parts, ability to write, evidence of muscle weakness
    B. Discuss alterations in sensation, proprioception, and impact on ability to do activities of daily living (ADLs)
    C. Discuss alternative strategies to prevent injury
      1. Instruct pt in safety measures and use of visual cues
      2. Encourage pt to take time to complete activities, focus attention to task
      3. Use potholder when cooking
      4. Use gloves when washing dishes, gardening
      5. Inspect skin for cuts, abrasions, burns daily, especially arms, legs, toes, fingers
    D. Refer as appropriate for occupational or physical therapy, diagnostic testing using EMG
    E. If pt presents with S/S of peripheral neuropathy, hold chemotherapy and discuss with physician

II. A. Assess pt's ability to perform ADLs such as eating, hygiene, dressing, walking, and handwriting
     B. Discuss and develop strategies to meet self-care needs
       1. Referral to occupational therapy for splint, etc.
       2. Involve family members in care planning
       3. Community resource referral as appropriate (homemaker, home health aide, visiting nurse)

III. A. Assess comfort level and presence of severe tingling or prickling sensation, cramping, or burning
     B. Assess intensity, quality, and frequency of discomfort
     C. Identify precipitating factors, such as warm or cold stimulation, and develop realistic plan to avoid precipitating factors
     D. Consider adjunctive analgesics with neurologic action for dysaesthetic pain: amitriptyline HCl (Elavil), phenytoin sodium (Dilantin)
     E. Consider nonpharmacologic intervention: teach pt guided imagery, progressive muscle relaxation, massage, etc.

Table 12 Standardized Nursing Care Plan for the
Patient Experiencing Neuropathy *Continued*

Nursing Diagnosis	Expected Outcome
IV. *Impaired mobility related to decreased proprioception, muscle dysfunction*	IV. A. Pt will ambulate safely
V. *Potential for sexual dysfunction related to altered tactile sensation, muscle weakness, changes in role*	V. A. Pt and significant other will identify alterations in sexual expression B. Pt and significant other will identify alternative methods of sexual expression
VI. *Potential for role change with changes and alterations in self-esteem and self-concept related to sensory/perceptual dysfunction, changes in social function, changes in ability to perform occupational role*	VI. A. Pt and family will demonstrate positive coping strategies
VII. *Potential for alteration in nutrition: less than body requirements related to taste distortions, anorexia, hypersensitivity to foods*	VII. A. Pt will eat balanced diet from four food groups B. Pt will attain ideal body weight following completion of treatment
VIII. *Potential for constipation related to autonomic neuropathy (vinca alkaloids)*	VIII. A. Pt will move bowels at least every other day

Nursing Intervention

IV. A. Assess pt's level of activity, muscle strength, and mobility level prior to chemotherapy, then prior to each treatment, and at each visit once therapy is completed
    B. Encourage pt to use visual cues to determine position of body parts
    C. Teach measures to prevent injury
    D. Refer for physical, occupational therapy, and assistive devices as needed

V. A. Discuss with pt the impact of treatment-related dysfunction on sexuality, social role, and self-esteem
    B. Discuss appropriate alternative means of sexual expression
    C. Refer for specific sexual counseling if diminished ability to have erection
    D. Observe for changes in needs related to affection and emotional support

VI. A. Assess impact of sensory/perceptual dysfunction on social and work roles: ability to meet role expectations of self and family
    B. Discuss modifications in job and role, as appropriate and available
    C. Refer pt to OT/PT to see if appliances available to foster rehabilitation (braces, etc.)
    D. Encourage independence and provide positive reinforcement for accomplishments
    E. Support pt as he or she grieves loss(es); assess need for support groups or counseling
    F. Support pt and family by providing information to help explain these behavioral responses to treatment-related dysfunction

VII. A. Assess dietary preferences, changes in food tolerances
     B. Teach pt to select high-calorie, high-protein foods
     C. Suggest dietary modifications based on taste changes (e.g., Crazy Jane Salt and spices if foods are tasteless)
     D. Perform periodic weights prior to each treatment cycle
     E. Evaluate pt's ability to do fine-motor movement to feed self, cook
     F. Refer to nutritionist or dietitian as needed
     G. Monitor laboratory values, especially magnesium and calcium, on cisplatin therapy

VIII. A. Assess normal elimination pattern
      B. Encourage pt to drink at least 3 liters of fluid/day
      C. Encourage daily exercise
      D. Teach pt to include bulky, high-fiber foods in diet
      E. Teach pt to self-administer stool softeners and laxatives as needed

Table 12 Standardized Nursing Care Plan for the
           Patient Experiencing Neuropathy *Continued*

Nursing Diagnosis	Expected Outcome
IX. *Knowledge deficit related to self-care measures related to neuropathic changes*	IX. A. Pt will identify risk of development of neuropathy B. Pt will identify signs and symptoms to report to health care provider

Sources: Ogrinc, M. (1985). Sensory/perceptual alterations related to peripheral neuropathy. In J. C. McNally, J. C. Stair, and E. T. Somerville (Eds.), *Guidelines for Cancer Nursing Practice,* Orlando, FL: Grune and Stratton, 185–188; Holden, S., and Felde, G. (1987). Nursing care of patients experiencing cisplatin-related peripheral neuropathies, *Oncology Nursing Forum, 14*(1): 13–19; Brager, B. L., and Yasko, J. M. (1984). *Care of the Client Receiving Chemotherapy.* Reston, VA: Reston Publishing Co.; Kaplan, R. S., and Wiernik, P. H. (1984). Neurotoxicity of antitumor agents. In M. C. Perry and J. W. Yarbro (Eds.), *Toxicity of Chemotherapy,* Orlando, FL: Grune and Stratton, 365–431.

Nursing Intervention

IX. A. Teach pt re potential side effect(s) of neuropathy
    1. Constipation
    2. Numbness/tingling in hands/feet
    3. Motor weakness
       a. Gait changes (e.g., foot drop)
       b. Loss of fine-motor movement (buttoning shirt, picking up dime)
    4. Inability of males to have erection
    5. Difficulty urinating
  B. Teach pt to report the occurrence of signs and symptoms of neuropathies

Table 13 Nursing Protocol for the Management of
Tumor Lysis Syndrome

Problem	Intervention
Fluid balance	Administer IV hydration. Monitor weight, I&O, response to diuretics. Observe for signs of fluid overload, especially patients with potential or preexisting cardiac damage.
Electrolyte balance	Monitor electrolytes q day or q 6–12 hrs as indicated. Correct imbalances as prescribed.
	Observe for signs of hyperkalemia: weakness, flaccid paralysis, EKG changes, cardiac arrest.
Potential renal failure	Monitor Ca^{++}, $PO4^+$, uric acid, BUN, and creatinine daily for the 5–7-day period of cytolysis.
	Maintain hydration, especially if preexisting renal insufficiency (creatinine $>$ 1.6 mg/dL, uric acid $\geq$ 8 mg/dL), and monitor urinary output.
	Administer allopurinol 300–800 mg PO q day.
	Monitor urine pH: maintain $\geq$ 7 by administering IV $NaHCO_3$ as prescribed.
	Report decreased urine output, lethargy.
	Prepare to manage patient on temporary hemodialysis if renal failure develops.
Potential effects of drug therapy	Observe for side effects from allopurinol: skin rashes, GI disturbances, fever (rarely), vasculitis, and blood dyscrasias.
	Decreased doses of 6-MP and azathioprine if given concurrently with allopurinol.
Potential cardiac irritability	Monitor lab values of increased K+ and decreased Ca^{++}.
	Check pulse rate and rhythm frequently. Report irregularity.
	Observe for EKG changes, cardiac arrest.
Potential neuromuscular irritability	Monitor serum Ca^{++} level.
	Observe for symptoms of hypocalcemia: tetany, positive Chvostek's and Trousseau's signs.

Source: Adapted from Moore, J. (1985). Metabolic emergencies: Tumor lysis syndrome. In B. L. Johnson and J. Gross (Eds.), *Handbook of Oncology Nursing,* New York: John Wiley and Sons, 470–476.

Ca^{++} = ionized calcium; K+ = ionized potassium; 6-MP = 6-mercaptopurine; $NaHCO_3$ = sodium bicarbonate; $PO4^+$ = phosphate ion(s).

Section II

Most Commonly Used Cancer Chemotherapeutic Drugs with Accompanying Care Plans

INTRODUCTION

Oncology nursing changes continually as the number and type of chemotherapeutic agents increases in unprecedented numbers. In working with the person who receives chemotherapy, these changes become more pronounced and demonstrate the type of information necessary for safe and effective clinical practice. Research and clinical experience broaden our understanding of treatment and the drug therapy that is required to care for patients safely.

Nursing process is the basis for nursing practice. It is solely the purview of nursing's domain. Nursing diagnosis is an integral part of the nursing process. This section integrates nursing process with chemotherapy administration.

Not all cancer chemotherapeutic agents from the companion textbook will be found in this handbook. Instead, we have chosen to include only the most commonly used agents in this newest edition of the handbook. In consultation with and with wise counsel from my colleague Reginald S. King, Pharm. D., B.C.O.P., oncology/bone marrow transplant clinical specialist and contributor to other books in the trifeminate chemotherapy series from Jones and Bartlett Publishers, we have made this selection. For additional information on chemotherapeutic agents not found in this book, we refer readers to *Cancer Chemotherapy: A Nursing Process Approach* by Barton-Burke, Wilkes, and Ingwersen, 3rd Edition, 2001.

The information in this book is not meant to replace any hospital formulary or manufacturer information. The authors and publisher of this book have made every effort to ensure that the dosage regimens set forth in the text are accurate and in accord with current labeling guidelines at the time of publication. However, in view of the constant flow of information resulting from ongoing research and clinical experience as well as changes in government regulations, nurses are urged to check the package insert of each drug they plan to administer to be certain that changes have not been made in its indications or contraindications or in the recommended dosage for each use. This is particularly important when a drug is new or infrequently employed.

Anastrozole
(Arimidex)

Class: Nonsteroidal aromatase inhibitor

MECHANISM OF ACTION

Inhibits the enzyme aromatase. Aromatase is one of the P-450 enzymes and is involved in estrogen biosynthesis. Circulating estrogen in post-menopausal women (mainly estradiol) arises from the aromatase-medi-ated conversion of androstenedione (made by the adrenals) to estrone, then estrone to estradiol, in the peripheral tissues, such as adipose tissue. Anastrozole is highly selective for this enzyme and does not affect steroid synthesis, so that estradiol synthesis is potently suppressed (to unde-tectable levels) while cortisol and aldosterone levels are unchanged.

METABOLISM

Extensively metabolized, with 85% of the drug metabolized by the liver. About 10% of the unchanged drug and 60% of the drug as metabo-lites are excreted in the urine within 72 hours of drug administration.

DOSAGE/RANGE

1 mg PO qd. No dosage adjustment required for mild to moderate hepatic impairment.

DRUG PREPARATION

None. Available as 1-mg tablet

DRUG ADMINISTRATION

Take orally with or without food, at approximately the same time daily

SPECIAL CONSIDERATIONS

Second-line therapy for postmenopausal women with advanced breast cancer.

Well-tolerated with low toxicity profile.

Coadministration of corticosteroids is not necessary.

Absolutely contraindicated during pregnancy.

Anastrozole

Nursing Diagnosis	Defining Characteristics
I. *Sexual dysfunction related to decreased estrogen levels*	I. A. Hot flashes (12%), asthenia or loss of energy (16%), and vaginal dryness may occur
II. *Potential alteration in cardiac output related to thrombophlebitis*	II. A. Thrombophlebitis may occur, but is uncommon
III. *Alteration in comfort related to headaches, weakness*	III. A. Headaches are mild and occur in about 13% of patients B. Decreased energy and weakness is common C. Mild swelling of arms/legs may occur and is mild
IV. *Potential alteration in nutrition, less than body requirements, related to nausea, diarrhea*	IV. A. Nausea is mild, with a 15% incidence. Diarrhea is uncommon and mild

Expected Outcomes	Nursing Interventions
I. A. Pt will verbalize understanding of the possibility of side effects affecting sexual function and strategies to cope with changes	I. A. As appropriate, explore with pt and partner patterns of sexuality and impact therapy may have B. Discuss strategies to preserve sexual health C. Teach pt that the vaginal dryness may be from menopause (and not the drug); she should avoid estrogen creams but use some lubrication
II. A. Cardiac output will remain at baseline	II. A. Identify pts at risk for thromboembolic complications B. Teach pts to report/come to emergency room for pain, redness, or marked swelling in arms or legs, or if shortness of breath or dizziness occur
III. A. Pt will report comfort throughout treatment process	III. A. Teach pt to take OTC analgesics for headache and to report headaches that are unrelieved by them B. Elevate extremities when at rest, as needed
IV. A. Pt will be without nausea or diarrhea	IV. A. Determine baseline weight, and monitor at each visit B. Teach pt about the possibility of nausea, and measures that may be used to alleviate it, including diet and dosing time C. Assess for changes in bowel pattern, and teach pt to report diarrhea D. Instruct pt in administration of antidiarrheal medications (Kaopectate, loperamide, etc.), and in reporting unrelieved diarrhea

Bicalutamide
(Casodex)

Class: Nonsteroidal antiandrogen

MECHANISM OF ACTION

Binds to androgen receptors in the prostate; affinity is four times greater than that of flutamide.

METABOLISM

Extensively metabolized in the liver. Decreased drug excretion in patients with moderate to severe hepatic dysfunction.

DOSAGE/RANGE

50 mg po qd

DRUG PREPARATION

None

DRUG ADMINISTRATION

Orally

SPECIAL CONSIDERATIONS

Use cautiously in patients with moderate to severe hepatic dysfunction.
Observe closely for toxicity, as dosage adjustment may be required.

No dose modification needed for renal dysfunction.

In a study comparing castration to bicalutamide 50 mg/day, there was no
difference in time to disease progression or subjective tolerance, but
overall health of group receiving castration was better.

Bicalutamide

Nursing Diagnosis	Defining Characteristics
I. *Alteration in comfort, related to gynecomastia and hot flashes*	I. A. Gynecomastia occurs in 23% of pts, breast tenderness in 26%, and hot flashes in 9.3%
II. *Alteration in nutrition, less than body requirements, related to nausea*	II. A. Nausea may occur in 6% of pts
III. *Alteration in elimination, related to constipation or diarrhea*	III. A. Incidence of constipation is 6%, while that of diarrhea is 2.5%

Expected Outcomes	Nursing Interventions
I. A. Pt will report comfort throughout treatment course	I. A. Teach pt about possibility of these side effects and discuss measures that may offer symptomatic reliefs
II. A. Pt will be without nausea	II. A. Teach pt that nausea may occur and to report it if it does B. Determine baseline weight and monitor at each visit C. Discuss strategies to minimize nausea, including diet modification and time of dosing
III. A. Pt will maintain baseline elimination pattern	III. A. Assess baseline elimination pattern B. Teach pt that alterations may occur and to report them if changes do not respond to OTC medications and dietary modifications

Bleomycin sulfate
(Blenoxane)

> *Class:* Antitumor antibiotic—isolated from fungus *Streptomyces verticullus*. Possesses both antitumor and antimicrobial actions.

MECHANISM OF ACTION

Primary action of bleomycin is to induce single-strand and double-strand breaks in DNA. DNA synthesis is inhibited. The action of drug is not exerted against RNA.

METABOLISM

Excreted via the renal system. About 70% is excreted unchanged in urine; 30–60 minutes after IV infusion, urine levels are 10 times the serum level.

DOSAGE/RANGE

5–20 U/m^2 once a week
10–20 U/m^2 twice a week
(frequency and schedule may vary according to protocol and age)

DRUG PREPARATION

Dilute powder in normal saline or sterile water.

DRUG ADMINISTRATION

IV, IM, or SC doses may be administered. Some clinical trials may utilize 24-hour infusions. There is a risk for anaphylaxis and hypotension with some diseases and with higher doses of drug. It may be recommended that a test dose be given before the first dose to detect hypersensitivity.

SPECIAL CONSIDERATIONS

Because of pulmonary toxicities with increasing dose, PFTs and CXR should be obtained before each course or as outlined by protocol.

Incidence of anaphylaxis increases over the age of 70.

May cause chemical fevers up to 103°–105°F, 39.5°–40.5°C (60%). May need to administer premedications such as acetaminophen, antihistamines, and in some cases steroids.

Watch for signs/symptoms of hypotension and anaphylaxis. Test dose needed.

May cause irritation at site of injection (is considered an irritant, not a vesicant).

Maximum cumulative lifetime dose: 400 U.

Decreases the oral bioavailability of digoxin when given together.

Decreases the pharmacologic effects of phenytoin when given in combination.

Bleomycin sulfate

Nursing Diagnosis	Defining Characteristics

I. *Potential alteration in comfort related to*
  A. Fever and chills
	I. A. 1. Fever and chills occur in 60% of pts 4–10 hrs after drug dose, persisting up to 24 hrs
	    2. Severity of reaction decreases with successive doses

B. Pain at tumor site	B. Pain at tumor site due to chemotherapy-induced cellular damage
II. *Potential for impaired skin integrity related to* A. Alopecia	II. A. Usually occurs late, 3–4 weeks after dose
B. Skin changes	B. Skin changes occur in 50% of pts (e.g., striae, pruritis, skin peeling—fingertips, hyperpigmentation, and hyperkeratosis)
C. Skin eruptions	C. Macular rash (hands and elbows), urticaria, and vesicles are the type of eruptions most likely to be seen

Expected Outcomes	Nursing Interventions
I. A. Pt will remain comfortable during therapy	I. A. 1. Assess pt for these symptoms during the hour following treatment 2. Discuss with MD premedication with acetaminophen, antihistamines, or steroids 3. Evaluate the effectiveness of the symptomatic relief that is prescribed 4. Monitor the quantity of cumulative dose
B. Pt will be supported during therapy	B. 1. Offer emotional support to pt 2. Reinforce information on the action and side effects of bleomycin 3. Discuss with MD medicating with acetaminophen
II. A. Pt will verbalize feelings re hair loss and identify strategies to cope with changes in body image	II. A. 1. Discuss with pt impact of hair loss 2. Suggest wig as appropriate prior to actual hair loss 3. Explore with pt response to actual hair loss and plan strategies to minimize distress (e.g., wig, scarf, cap)
B. 1. Skin discomfort will be minimized and skin will remain intact 2. Pt will verbalize feelings re skin changes	B. 1. Skin changes are not an indication to stop the drug 2. Discuss with MD symptomatic management of skin changes 3. Reinforce pt teaching on the action and side effects of bleomycin 4. Offer emotional support
C. 1. Skin discomfort will be minimized, and skin will remain intact 2. Pt will verbalize feelings re skin changes	C. 1. Skin eruptions are not an indication to stop the drug 2. Discuss with MD symptomatic management

Bleomycin sulfate *Continued*

Nursing Diagnosis	Defining Characteristics
D. Nail changes	D. Nail changes and possible nail loss can occur
III. *Potential alteration in nutrition related to* A. Nausea and vomiting	III. A. Nausea and vomiting are rare
B. Anorexia and weight loss	B. Anorexia and weight loss may occur and may be prolonged
C. Stomatitis	C. Stomatitis may decrease ability and desire to eat

IV. *Potential for impaired gas exchange related to pulmonary toxicity*	IV. A. Incidence 8–10%: pneumonitis (rales, dyspn infiltrate) may progress to irreversible pulmonary fibrosis; PFTs decrease before X-changes
	B. High risk
	  1. Age > 70 years old
	  2. Dose > 150 U (maximum lifetime dose i 400 U)
	  3. XRT to chest (prior to chemotherapy or concomitantly)

Expected Outcomes	Nursing Interventions
	3. Reinforce pt teaching on the action and side effects of bleomycin
	4. Offer emotional support
D. Pt will verbalize feelings about nail changes and idenify strategies to cope wtih loss	D. 1. Nail changes are not an indication to stop the drug
	2. Discuss with MD symptomatic management
	3. Reinforce pt teaching on the action and side effects of bleomycin
	4. Offer emotional support
III. A. Pt will be without nausea and vomiting; if either occurs, it will be minimal	III. A. 1. Premedicate with antiemetic if needed and continue prophylactically to prevent nausea and vomiting
	2. Encourage small, frequent feedings of favorite foods, especially high-calorie, high-protein foods
B. Pt will maintain baseline weight ± 5%	B. 1. Encourage small, frequent feedings of favorite foods, especially high-calorie, high-protein foods
	2. Encourage use of spices
	3. Weekly weights
C. Oral mucous membranes will remain intact and without infection	C. 1. Teach pt oral assessment
	2. Encourage pt to report early stomatitis
	3. Teach pt oral hygiene
	4. Medicate for pain as needed
IV. A. Early s/s or pulmonary toxicity will be identified	IV. A. Discuss with MD the need for pulmonary function tests and CXR prior to beginning therapy
	B. Assess lung sounds prior to drug administration
	C. Instruct pt to report cough, dyspnea, shortness of breath

Bleomycin sulfate *Continued*

Nursing Diagnosis	Defining Characteristics
V. *Potential for sexual dysfunction*	V. A. Drug is mutagenic and probably teratogenic
VI. *Potential for injury related to anaphylaxis*	VI. A. 1% of lymphoma pts experience anaphylaxis
	B. S/s include tachycardia, wheezing, hypotension, facial edema

Expected Outcomes	Nursing Interventions
V. A. Pt and significant other will understand needs for contraception B. Pt and significant other will identify strategies to cope with sexual dysfunction	V. A. 1. As appropriate, explore with pt and significant other issues of reproductive and sexuality pattern and impact chemotherapy may have on them 2. Discuss strategies to preserve sexual and reproductive health (e.g., sperm banking, contraception)
VI. A. Early s/s of hypersensitivity will be identified	VI. A. Review standing orders for management of pt in anaphylaxis and identify location of anaphylaxis kit containing ephinephrine 1:1000, hydrocortisone sodium succinate (Solucortef), diphenhydramine HCL (Benadryl), Aminophylline, H_2 blockers, and others B. Prior to drug administration, obtain baseline vital signs and record mental status C. Observe for following s/s during infusion, usually occurring within first 15 mins of start of infusion: 1. *Subjective* a. Generalized itching b. Nausea c. Chest tightness d. Crampy abdominal pain e. Difficulty speaking f. Anxiety g. Agitation h. Sense of impending doom i. Uneasiness j. Desire to urinate or defecate k. Dizziness l. Chills 2. *Objective* a. Flushed appearance (angioedema of face, neck, eyelids, hands, feet) b. Localized or generalized urticaria

Bleomycin sulfate *Continued*

Nursing Diagnosis	Defining Characteristics
VI. *Potential for injury related to anaphylaxis*	B. S/s include tachycardia, wheezing, hypotension, facial edema

Expected Outcomes	Nursing Interventions

	c. Respiratory distress ± wheezing
	    d. Hypotension
	    e. Cyanosis
	D. If reaction occurs, stop infusion and notify MD
	E. Place pt in supine position to promote perfusion of visceral organs
	F. Monitor vital signs until stable
	G. Provide emotional reassurance to pt and family
	H. Maintain pt airway and have CPR equipment ready if needed
	I. Document incident
	J. Discuss with MD desensitization versus drug discontinuance for further dosing

Busulfan
(Myleran)

Class: Alkylating agent

MECHANISM OF ACTION

Forms carbonium ions through the release of a methane sulfonate group. This results in the alkylating of DNA. Acts primarily on granulocyte precursors in the bone marrow and is cell cycle phase-nonspecific.

METABOLISM

Well absorbed orally; almost all metabolites are excreted in the urine. Has a very short half-life.

DOSAGE/RANGE

2–10 mg/day po for 2–3 weeks initially, then maintenance dose of 2–6 mg/m^2 po qd or 0.05 mg/kg po qd. Dose titrated to WBC counts.

DRUG PREPARATION

None

DRUG ADMINISTRATION

Available in 2-mg scored tablets given po.

SPECIAL CONSIDERATIONS

If WBC is high, patient is at risk for hyperuricemia. Allopurinol and hydration may be indicated.

Follow weekly CBC and platelet count initially, then monthly. Dose is decreased to maintenance when leukocyte count falls below 50,000 mm^3.

Hyperpigmentation of skin creases may occur due to increased melanin production.

If given according to accepted guidelines, patient should have minimal side effects.

Busulfan

Nursing Diagnosis	Defining Characteristics

I.   *Potential for infection*
   A. Myelosuppression
   B. Delayed, refractory pancytopenia
	I. A. Nadir 11–30 days, with recovery occurring over 24–54 days
	   B. Delayed, refractory pancytopenia has occurred

II. *Potential for impaired gas exchange related to interstitial pulmonary fibrosis (rare)*	II. A. Rare complication; may occur within a year of beginning therapy, but usually occurs after long-term therapy
	   B. Symptoms may be delayed and usually occur after 4 years: anorexia, cough, rales, dyspnea, fever
	   C. Usually fatal due to rapid diffuse fibrosis; high-dose corticosteroids may be helpful

III. *Potential for sexual dysfunction*	III. A. Testicular atrophy, impotence, and amenorrhea may occur
	   B. Successful pregnancies have been described after and during treatment with busulfan
	   C. Men may experience gynecomastia
	   D. Drug is potentially teratogenic

Expected Outcomes	**Nursing Interventions**
I. A. Pt will have normal recovery of bone marrow function B. Pt will be without infection, bleeding	I. A. Monitor CBC weekly initially, then at least monthly B. Monitor WBC closely: drug dose adjustment or discontinuance is based on WBC

II. A. Pulmonary dysfunction will be identified early	II. A. Carefully assess pulmonary function of pts receiving long-term therapy
	   1. Breath sounds and presence of dyspnea
	   2. Periodic pulmonary function studies
	B. Assess for underlying conditions (opportunistic infections, leukemic infiltrates)
	C. Lung biopsy may be needed to diagnose "busulfan lung"; drug should be stopped *immediately* if this occurs

III. A. Pt will understand potential dysfunction and that sterility may occur B. Pt and significant other will discuss potential impact of sterility on their lives C. Pt will understand importance of birth control if appropriate	III. A. Prechemo assessment of sexual patterns and function; institute pt and significant other teaching B. Facilitate discussion between pt and partner re reproductive issues. Provide information, support counseling, and referral as needed C. As appropriate, discuss birth control measures

Busulfan injection
(Busulfex)

Class: Alkylating agent

MECHANISM OF ACTION

Forms carbonium ions through the release of a methane sulfonate group.
This results in the alkylating of DNA. Acts primarily on granulocyte
precursors in the bone marrow and is cell cycle phase-nonspecific.

METABOLISM

Thirty percent of drug is excreted in the urine over 48 hours; negligible
amounts have been recovered in feces.

DOSAGE/RANGE

0.8 mg/kg of ideal body weight (IBW) or actual body weight (whichever
is lower) q 6 hours as a 2-hour infusion for a total of 16 doses, followed by cytoxan.

DRUG PREPARATION

Dilute with NS or D_5W.

Diluent quantity should be ten times the volume of Busulfex so that the
final concentration of the drug is 0.5 mg/ml.

Open ampule, withdraw drug using the filter needle provided, remove
the needle, and inject the drug into the IV bag, which already contains the correct amount of fluid.

DRUG ADMINISTRATION

Administer using an IV pump over 2 hours.

When mixed in NS, is stable (refrigerated) for 12 hours. In D_5W, is stable at room temperature for 8 hours. Infusion must be completed within these 2 time frames.

SPECIAL CONSIDERATIONS

Profound myelosuppression occurs in all patients. Drug is currently indicated ONLY for patients who are getting conditioning regimen for hematopoetic progenitor cell transplantation.

Diluted drug must be used within 8 (if mixed in D_5W) or 12 (if mixed in NS) hours of reconstitution.

Crosses the blood-brain barrier. Patients should be premedicated with phenytoin before drug administration.

Probable increased risk of hepatic veno-occlusive disease with patients who have history of XRT or greater than 3 cycles of chemotherapy or prior progenitor cell transplantation. Elevated LFTs are common.

Busulfan injection

Nursing Diagnosis	Defining Characteristics
I. *Alteration in cardiac output*	I. A. Mild to moderate tachycardia noted in 50% of patients; various other rhythm abnormalities occurred in less than 10% of patients B. Mild to moderate thrombosis, usually associated with central venous catheter C. Hypertension noted in 25% of pts D. Vasodilation occurred in 23% of pts, with 17% experiencing hypotension
II. *Infection and bleeding related to bone marrow depression*	II. A. At the indicated doses, busulfan injection produces profound myelosuppression in all pts. Severe leukopenia occurs in 100% of pts, thrombocytopenia in 86%, and anemia in 50% of pts
III. *Alteration in nutrition related to GI disturbances*	III. A. Mild to moderate nausea/vomiting occurs in greater than 90% of patients B. Stomatitis common; is mild–moderate in most pts, but severe in 13% of patients C. Hyperglycemia occurs in over half of pts D. Anorexia and dyspepsia common, usually mild–moderate in severity E. Diarrhea and constipation both occur

Expected Outcomes	Nursing Interventions
I. A. Patient will maintain baseline cardiac function B. Changes in cardiac function will be identified early	I. A. Assess baseline cardiac status, including HR, BP, EKG, etc. B. Monitor pt for changes in cardiac parameters throughout treatment course; report changes C. Monitor central venous lines for patency; watch for symptoms of venous thrombosis
II. A. Pt will be without s/s of infection or bleeding B. Signs of infection and/or bleeding will be identified, reported, and treated early	II. A. Monitor Hct, WBC with differential, and platelets prior to drug administration. Discuss any abnormalities with physician B. Monitor continuously for s/s of infection and bleeding, instruct patient in self-assessment and to report s/s immediately C. Teach pt self-care measures to minimize risk of infection and bleeding, including avoidance of OTC aspirin-containing medications D. Monitor CBC at least daily (more often if s/s of bleeding occur)—transfuse with PRBCs and platelets per protocol and physician order
III. A. Pt will be without nausea or vomiting B. Nausea/vomiting will be minimized C. Serum glucose will remain within normal limits D. Pt will maintain weight within 5% of baseline E. Pt will maintain baseline patterns of elimination	III. A. Premedicate with antiemetics and continue for 24 hrs to prevent nausea and vomiting B. Encourage small, frequent feedings of cool, bland foods and liquids C. Instruct pt in oral self-care measures, and to report nausea/vomiting to health care providers D. Weigh pt each day. Dietary consult prior to treatment to determine pt preferences and educate pt in low-bacteria diet E. Follow serum glucose; report abnormal values

Busulfan injection *Continued*

Nursing Diagnosis	Defining Characteristics
III. *Alteration in nutrition related to GI disturbances*	
IV. *Potential for impaired gas exchange related to pulmonary toxicities*	IV. A. Dyspnea occurs in 22% of pts B. Mild/moderate rhinitis and cough observed in 44% of pts C. Less frequent side effects include hyperventilation, respiratory failure, alveolar hemorrhages, asthma, pleural effusion, and hypoxia
V. *Alteration in comfort related to neurologic toxicities*	V. A. Anxiety and insomnia occur frequently B. Mild/moderate headache occurs in 65% of pts, unspecified pain in 40% C. Dizziness and depression noted in over 20% of pts D. Less frequent side effects, occurring in less than 10% of pts, include nervousness, delirium, agitation
VI. *Alteration in skin integrity related to rash*	VI. A. 50% of pts experience mild/moderate rash, 29% pruritis

Expected Outcomes	Nursing Interventions
	F. Monitor bowel elimination pattern: use dietary measures, antidiarrheals or laxatives to maintain pts baseline pattern
IV. A. Pt will maintain pulmonary function within baseline limits B. Pulmonary side effects will be identified and treated early	IV. A. Assess baseline pulmonary function B. Monitor pt throughout treatment course for objective and subjective changes in breathing and lung sounds C. Assess for underlying conditions (infection, effusions, leukemic infiltrates) D. Report changes in pulmonary function
V. A. Pt will report relative comfort, adequate coping throughout treatment	V. A. Explain to pt that neurologic toxicities may occur, to report discomfort and changes in neuro functioning B. Medicate for symptoms above, report all changes C. Relaxation/meditation as able
VI. A. Pt's skin will remain intact throughout treatment course	VI. A. Assess pt q day for changes in skin B. Inform pt about possibility of skin changes, to report them when they occur C. Topical agents as ordered, antipruritic agents as needed

Capecitabine
(Xeloda, N4-pentoxycarbonyl-5-deoxy-5-fluorocytidine)

Class: Fluoropyrimidine carbamate

MECHANISM OF ACTION

Metabolites bind to thymidylate synthetase, inhibiting the formation of uracil from thymidylate, and reducing the cell's ability to produce DNA. It also prevents cell division by hindering the formation of RNA, by causing nuclear transcription enzymes to mistakenly incorporate its metabolites in the process of RNA transcription.

METABOLISM

Absorbed from the intestinal mucosa as an intact molecule, metabolized in the liver to intermediary metabolite, and then in the liver and tumor tissue to 5-FU precursor. It is then converted through catalytic activation to 5-FU at the tumor site. Metabolites are cleared in the urine.

DOSAGE/RANGE

2500 mg/m^2 po in two divided doses with food for 2 weeks. Treatment followed by a 1-week rest period. Treatment repeated every 3 weeks.

PREPARATION/ADMINISTRATION

Oral

Administer after meals with plenty of water.

Divide daily dose in half; take 12 hours apart.

SPECIAL CONSIDERATIONS

Monitor bilirubin baseline and before each cycle, as dose modifications
   are necessary with hyperbilirubinemia.

Folic acid should be avoided while taking drug.

Capecitabine

Nursing Diagnosis	Defining Characteristics
I. *Potential for infection and bleeding related to bone marrow depression*	I. A. Commonly causes anemia, neutropenia, and thrombocytopenia
II. *Altered nutrition, less than body requirements, related to nausea and vomiting, stomatitis, and diarrhea*	II. A. Nausea and vomiting occur in 30–50% of pts B. Stomatitis and diarrhea also occur in about 50% of pts
III. *Alteration in skin integrity/ comfort related to hand/ foot syndrome*	III. A. Hand/foot syndrome occurs in more than h of pts and is characterized by tingling, numbness, pain, erythema, dryness, rash, swelling, and/or pruritus of hands and feet

Expected Outcomes	Nursing Interventions
I. A. Pt will be without s/s of infection or bleeding B. Signs of infection and/or bleeding will be identified and reported early	I. A. Monitor Hct, WBC with differential, and platelets prior to drug administration; discuss any abnormalities with physician B. Assess for s/s infection and bleeding, and instruct pt in self-assessment and to report s/s immediately C. Teach pt self-care measures to minimize risk of infection and bleeding, including avoidance of OTC aspirin-containing medications
II. A. Pt will be without nausea, vomiting, stomatitis, and diarrhea	II. A. Premedicate with antiemetics and continue for 24 hrs to prevent nausea and vomiting B. Encourage small, frequent feedings of cool, bland foods and liquids C. Instruct pt in oral self-care measures, and to report nausea/vomiting to health care providers
III. Pt will verbalize understanding of informing physician if hand/foot syndrome occurs	III. Teach pt about the possibility of this side effect, and to inform physician immediately should it occur

Carboplatin
(Paraplatin)

Class: Alkylating agent (heavy metal complex)

MECHANISM OF ACTION

A second-generation platinum analog. The cytotoxicity is identical to that of the parent, *Cis*-platinum. Cell cycle phase nonspecific. Reacts with nucleophilic sites on DNA, causing predominantly intrastrand and interstrand cross-links rather than DNA-protein cross-links. These cross-links are similar to those formed with *Cis*-platinum but are formed later.

METABOLISM

At 24 hours post-administration, approximately 70% of carboplatin is excreted in the urine. The mean half-life is roughly 100 minutes.

DOSAGE/RANGE

As a single agent, 360 mg/m^2 on day 1, cycle repeated every 4 weeks; *or* 300 mg/m^2 on day 1 combined with cyclophosphamide for advanced ovarian cancer, cycle repeated every 4 weeks. Drug administration may have to be delayed if neutrophil count is less than 2000 mm^3 or platelet count is less than 100,000 mm^3.

Drug dose reduction for urine creatinine clearance < 60 ml/minute. Since carboplatin has predictable pharmacokinetics based on the drug's excretion by the kidneys, area under the curve (AUC) dosing is now recommended for this drug. The Calvert formula is used where the total dose (mg) = (target AUC) × (glomerular filtration rate [GFR] + 25). The GFR is approximated by the urine creatinine clearance, either estimated or actual. AUC dose is determined by the physician based on the treatment plan, and for previously treated patients receiving single-agent carboplatin, is 4–6 mg/ml/min (see package insert).

DRUG PREPARATION

Available as a white powder in amber vial.

Reconstitute with sterile water for injection, D_5W, or NS.

Dilute further in D_5W or normal saline.

The solution is chemically stable for 24 hours; discard solution after 8 hours because of the lack of bacteriostatic preservative.

DRUG ADMINISTRATION

Administered by IV bolus over 30 minutes to 1 hour.

May also be given as a continuous infusion over 24 hours.

SPECIAL CONSIDERATIONS

Does not have the renal toxicity seen with *Cis*-platinum.

Monitor urine creatinine clearance.

Carboplatin

Nursing Diagnosis	Defining Characteristics
I. *Potential for infection and bleeding related to bone marrow depression*	I. A. Myelosuppression is major dose-limiting toxicity B. Thrombocytopenia nadir 14–21 days, with recovery by day 28 C. Leukopenia nadir usually follows thrombocytopenia by 1 week but may take 5–6 weeks to recover D. Mild anemia frequently observed
II. *Altered nutrition, less than body requirements related to* A. Nausea and vomiting	II. A. 1. Nausea and vomiting begin 6+ hrs after dose and usually last for < 24 hrs 2. 80% of pts experience some nausea or vomiting but often mild to moderate in severity
B. Anorexia	B. Somewhat common but usually lasts for less than 1 day
C. Stomatitis	C. Occurs in ~10% of pts but usually mild
D. Diarrhea	D. Occurs in ~10% of pts but is usually mild
E. Hepatic dysfunction	E. Mild to moderate reversible disturbances in liver function studies, especially alkaline phosphatase and SGOT, rarely SGPT and bilirubin

Expected Outcomes	Nursing Interventions
A. Pt will be without s/s of infection or bleeding B. S/s of infection or bleeding will be identified early	I. A. Monitor CBC, platelet count prior to drug administration, as well as s/s of infection or bleeding B. Instruct pt in self-assessment of s/s of infection or bleeding C. Dose reduction often necessary (35–50%) if bone marrow function is compromised
II. A. 1. Pt will be without nausea and vomiting 2. Nausea and vomiting, should they occur, will be minimal B. Pt will maintain baseline weight ± 5% C. Oral mucous membranes will remain intact and without infection D. Pt will have minimal diarrhea E. Hepatic dysfunction will be identified early	II. A. 1. Premedicate with antiemetics and continue prophylactically × 24 hrs to prevent nausea and vomiting 2. Encourage small, frequent feedings of cool, bland foods and liquids 3. If vomiting occurs, assess for s/s of fluid/electrolyte imbalance: monitor I&O, daily weights, lab results B. 1. Encourage small, frequent feedings of favorite foods, especially high-calorie, high-protein foods 2. Encourage use of spices 3. Weekly weights 4. Dietary consult as needed C. 1. Teach pt oral assessment and oral hygiene regimen 2. Encourage pt to report early stomatitis D. 1. Encourage pt to report onset of diarrhea 2. Administer or teach pt to self-administer antidiarrheal medications E. 1. Monitor LFTs (i.e., alkaline phosphatase, SGOT, SGPT, and bilirubin) periodically during treatment 2. Monitor pt for any elevations in LFTs 3. Dose modifications may be necessary if elevation occurs

Carboplatin *Continued*

Nursing Diagnosis	Defining Characteristics
III. *Altered urinary elimination related to nephrotoxicity*	III. A. Does not have the renal toxicity seen with Cis-platinum B. Minimal diuresis and hydration needed; if occurs, usually mild
IV. *Potential for sensory/perceptual alterations due to high-dose carboplatin*	IV. A. Neurotoxicity and ototoxicity rare; similar to those seen with Cis-platinum (but not as severe) B. Neurotoxicity: peripheral neuropathies, reversible confusion and dementia C. Ototoxicity: transient
V. *Potential for sexual dysfunction*	V. A. Drug is mutagenic and probably teratogenic
VI. *Potential for injury related to hypersensitivity reactions*	VI. A. Anaphylaxis or anaphylactic-like reactions have been reported (reactions similar to parent drug cisplatin) 1. Tachycardia 2. Wheezing 3. Hypotension 4. Facial edema B. Occurs within a few minutes of initiating the drug and usually responds to steroid, epinephrine, or antihistamines

Expected Outcomes	Nursing Interventions
III. A. Pt will be without renal dysfunction B. Early s/s of renal dysfunction will be identified	III. A. Monitor BUN and creatinine prior to initiating drug administration, as drug is excreted by the kidneys B. Check parameters of BUN and creatinine established in protocol, as myelotoxicity is directly related to renal function status C. Dose modifications may be made for renal impairment based on urine creatinine clearance
IV. A. Neuropathies and ototoxicities will be identified early	IV. A. If pt is to receive high-dose carboplatin, obtain baseline neurological and auditory test B. Assess pt for changes during treatment course C. Teach pt the potential for neurologic toxicity problems and to report any changes
V. A. Pt and significant other will understand needs for contraception B. Pt and significant other will identify strategies to cope with sexual dysfunction	V. A. As appropriate, explore with pt and significant other issues of reproductive and sexuality pattern and impact chemotherapy will have B. Discuss strategies to preserve sexual and reproductive health (sperm banking, contraception)
VI. A. Early s/s of hypersensitivity will be identified	VI. A. Teach pt about the potential of a hypersensitivity reaction and ask pt to report any unusual s/s B. Assess baseline mental status C. Adverse reaction kit with epinephrine in room D. If reaction occurs, administer treatment per MD orders E. Document anaphylactic incident F. Discuss with MD precautionary measures to be taken before next drug dose is given *or* drug discontinuance

Carmustine
(BiCNU, BCNU)

Class: Nitrosoureas

MECHANISM OF ACTION

Alkylates DNA in the same manner as classic mustard agents—by causing cross-strand breaks. Also, carbamoylates cellular proteins of nucleic acid synthesis. Is cell cycle phase-nonspecific.

METABOLISM

Rapidly distributed and metabolized, with a plasma half-life of 1 hour; 70% of IV dose is excreted in urine within 96 hours. Significant concentrations of drug remain in CSF for 9 hours due to lipid solubility of drug.

DOSAGE/RANGE

75–100 mg/m^2 IV/day $\times$ 2 days
  or
200–225 mg/m^2 every 6 weeks
  or
40 mg/m^2 day on 5 successive days

DRUG PREPARATION

Add sterile alcohol (provided with drug) to vial, then add sterile water for injection.
May be further diluted with 100–250 ml D$_5$W or NS.

DRUG ADMINISTRATION

Discard solution 2 hours after mixing.

Administer via volutrol over 45–120 minutes as tolerated by patient.

SPECIAL CONSIDERATIONS

Drug is an irritant; avoid extravasation.

Pain at the injection site or along the vein is common. Treat by applying ice pack above the injection site and decreasing the infusion flow rate.

Patient may act inebriated due to the alcohol diluent and may experience flushing.

Increased myelosuppression when given with cimetidine.

Can decrease the pharmacologic effects of phenytoin.

Carmustine

Nursing Diagnosis	Defining Characteristics
I. *Potential for infection related to myelosuppression*	I. A. Nadir: 3–5 weeks after dose, persists 1–3 weeks longer B. Myelosuppression is cumulative and may be delayed
II. *Alteration in comfort related to drug administration* A. Pain along vein B. Flushing of skin or burning of eyes	II. A. 1. Drug diluent is absolute alcohol 2. Drug is an irritant and can cause pain along a vein 3. True thrombophlebitis is rare 4. Venospasms commonly occur during rapid infusion B. Occurs with rapid drug infusion
III. *Altered nutrition, less than body requirements related to* A. Nausea and vomiting B. Liver dysfunction (rare) related to subacute hepatitis	III. A. Severe nausea and vomiting may occur 2 hrs after administration and last 4–6 hrs B. Abnormal SGOT, alkaline phosphatase, and serum bilirubin have occurred; also painless jaundice and hepatic coma, usually reversible
IV. *Altered urinary elimination related to nephrotoxicity*	IV. A. Increased BUN occurs in ~10% of treated pts, usually reversible

Expected Outcomes	**Nursing Interventions**
I. A. Pt will be without infection	I. A. Monitor CBC, including WBC differential, prior to drug administration
B. Early s/s of infection will be identified	B. Drug dosage may be reduced or held for lower than normal blood values
II. A. Pt will be without pain or will have minimal discomfort during infusion	II. A. 1. Administer drug in 100–250 ml D_5W or NS over 45–120 mins 2. Use ice pack above injection site, decrease infusion rate, further dilute drug if pain occurs
B. Pt will be without flushing or burning of eyes	B. Administer drug slowly; if symptoms occur, slow rate of infusion
III. A. 1. Pt will be without nausea and vomiting 2. Nausea and vomiting, if they occur, will be minimal	III. A. 1. Premedicate with antiemetics and continue prophylactically × 24 hrs to prevent nausea and vomiting, at least for first treatment 2. Encourage small, frequent feedings of cool, bland foods and liquids
B. Laboratory abnormalities will be identified early	B. 1. Monitor LFTs (SGOT, SGPT, LDH, alkaline phosphatase, bilirubin) during treatment 2. Notify MD of elevations
IV. A. Pt will be without renal dysfunction	IV. A. Monitor BUN and creatinine prior to initiating drug dose, as drug is excreted by the kidneys
B. Early s/s of renal dysfunction will be identified	B. Check parameters of BUN and creatinine established in protocol, as myelotoxicity is directly related to renal function C. Dose modifications may need to be made for renal impairment

Carmustine *Continued*

Nursing Diagnosis	Defining Characteristics
V. *Potential for impaired gas exchange related to pulmonary fibrosis*	V. A. Presents as insidious cough and dyspnea or sudden onset of respiratory failure
	B. CXR shows interstitial infiltrates
	C. Pulmonary function tests show hypoxia with diffusion and restrictive defects
	D. Risk may increase with concurrent cyclophosphamide
	E. Risk increases as dose exceeds gm/m^2
	F. Incidence 20–30% with mortality of 24–80%
VI. *Potential for sexual dysfunction*	VI. A. Drug is teratogenic

Expected Outcomes	Nursing Interventions

V. A. Early dysfunction will be identified	V. A. Assess pts at risk
	  1. Cumulative dose 1 gm/m^2
	  2. Preexisting lung disease
	  3. Concurrent cyclophosphamide therapy or thoracic irradiation
	B. Assess breath sounds and presence of dyspnea
	C. Monitor pulmonary function studies periodically for evidence of pulmonary dysfunction

VI. A. Pt and significant other understand need for contraception	VI. A. 1. As appropriate, explore with pt and significant other issues of reproductive and sexuality pattern and impact chemotherapy may have 2. Discuss strategies to preserve sexual and reproductive health (e.g., sperm banking, contraception)

Chlorambucil
(Leukeran)

Class: Alkylating agent

MECHANISM OF ACTION

Alkylates DNA by causing strand breaks and crosslinks in the DNA. Is a derivative of a nitrogen mustard.

METABOLISM

Pharmacokinetics are poorly understood. Is well absorbed orally, with a plasma half-life of 1.5 hours. Degradation is slow; appears to be eliminated by metabolic transformation with 60% of drug excreted in urine in 24 hours.

DOSAGE/RANGE

0.1–0.2 mg/kg/day (equals 4–8 mg/m^2/day) to initiate treatment
  or
14 mg/m^2/day $\times$ 5 days with a repeat every 21–28 days depending upon platelet count and WBC

DRUG PREPARATION

None

DRUG ADMINISTRATION

Oral

SPECIAL CONSIDERATIONS

Simultaneous administration of barbiturates may increase toxicity of
chlorambucil due to hepatic drug activation.

Chlorambucil

Nursing Diagnosis	Defining Characteristics
I. *Potential for infection related to myelosuppression*	I. A. WBC decreases for 10 days after last dose
	B. Neutropenia, thrombocytopenia occur with prolonged use and may be irreversible
	C. Secondary malignancies have been reported (acute myelogenous leukemia)
	D. Increased toxicity may occur with prior barbiturate use
II. *Potential for sexual dysfunction*	II. A. Drug is mutagenic and teratogenic and suppresses gonadal function, with consequent sterility (permanent or temporary)
	B. Amenorrhea
	C. Oligospermia
III. *Potential alteration in nutrition related to* A. Nausea and vomiting	III. A. Nausea and vomiting are rare
B. Anorexia and weight loss	B. Anorexia and weight loss may occur and be prolonged
C. Hepatic dysfunction	C. Hepatitis is rare but may occur (also disturbances in liver function)

Expected Outcomes	Nursing Interventions
I. A. Pt will be without infection B. Early s/s of infection will be identified	I. A. Monitor CBC, including WBC differential, prior to drug administration B. Drug dosage may be reduced or held for lower than normal blood values
II. A. Pt and significant other will understand need for contraception B. Pt and significant other will discuss strategies to cope with change in sexual function	II. A. As appropriate, explore with pt and significant other issues of reproductive and sexuality pattern and impact chemotherapy will have B. Discuss strategies to preserve sexual and reproductive health (e.g., sperm banking, contraception)
III. A. 1. Pt will be without nausea and vomiting 2. If they occur, they are minimal B. Pt will maintain baseline weight ± 5% C. Hepatic dysfunction will be identified early	III. A. 1. Premedicate with antiemetic if ordered and continue prophylactically to prevent nausea and vomiting 2. Encourage small, frequent feedings of cool, bland foods and liquids 3. Administer oral dose on an empty stomach B. 1. Encourage small, frequent feedings of favorite foods, especially high-calorie, high-protein foods 2. Encourage use of spices 3. Weekly weights C. 1. Monitor LFTs (i.e., alkaline phosphatase and bilirubin) periodically during treatment 2. Monitor pt for any elevations 3. Dose modifications may be necessary if elevation occurs

Chlorambucil *Continued*

Nursing Diagnosis	Defining Characteristics
IV. *Potential for impaired skin integrity*	IV. A. Dermatitis and urticaria may occur (rarely) B. Cross-hypersensitivity may exist between Alkeran and chlorambucil (skin rash)
V. *Potential for impaired gas exchange related to pulmonary fibrosis*	V. A. Alveolar dysplasia and pulmonary fibrosis may occur with long-term use B. Infrequent
VI. *Potential for sensory/ perceptual alterations (rare)*	VI. A. Ocular disturbances may occur 1. Diplopia 2. Papilledema 3. Retinal hemorrhage

Expected Outcomes	Nursing Interventions

IV. A. Skin will remain intact
     B. Early skin impairment will be identified
	IV. A. 1. Assess skin for integrity
	          2. If symptoms are severe, discuss drug discontinuance with MD

V. A. Early dysfunction will be identified	V. A. Assess pts at risk
	          1. Cumulative dose 1 gm/m^2
	          2. Preexisting lung disease
	          3. Concurrent cyclophosphamide or thoracic irradiation
	     B. Assess breath sounds and presence of dyspnea
	     C. Monitor pulmonary function studies periodically for evidence of pulmonary dysfunction

VI. A. Visual disturbances will be identified early	VI. A. Assess vision before giving treatment B. Encourage pt to report any visual changes

Cisplatin
(*Cis*-Platinum, CDDP, Platinum, Platinol)

Class: Heavy metal that acts like alkylating agent

MECHANISM OF ACTION

Inhibits DNA synthesis by forming interstrand and intrastrand cross-links and by denaturing the double helix, preventing cell replication. Is cell cycle phase-nonspecific. Has chemical properties similar to that of bifunctional alkylating agents.

METABOLISM

Rapidly distributed to tissues (predominantly the liver and kidneys), with less than 10% in plasma 1 hour after infusion. Clearance from plasma proceeds slowly after the first 2 hours due to platinum's covalent bonding with serum proteins; 20–74% of administered drug is excreted in the urine within 24 hours.

DOSAGE/RANGE

50–120 mg/m^2 every 3–4 weeks
   or
15–20 mg/m^2 × 5 repeated every 3–4 weeks

DRUG PREPARATION

10-mg and 50-mg vials. Add sterile water to develop a concentration of 1 mg/ml.

Further dilute solution with 250 ml or more of NS or D_5W $^1/_2$ NS. Never mix with D_5W, as a precipitate will form.

Refrigerate lyophilized drug, but *not* reconstituted drug, as a precipitate will form.

DRUG ADMINISTRATION

Avoid aluminum needles when administering, as precipitate will form.

SPECIAL CONSIDERATIONS

Hydrate vigorously before and after administering drug. Urine output should be at least 100–150 ml/hr. Mannitol or furosemide diuresis may be needed to ensure this output.

Hypersensitivity reactions have occurred, manifested by wheezing, flushing, hypotension, tachycardia. Usually occur within minutes of starting infusion. Treat with epinephrine, corticosteroids, antihistamines.

Decreases the pharmacologic effects of phenytoin.

Cisplatin

Nursing Diagnosis	Defining Characteristics
I. *Potential alteration in urinary elimination*	I. A. Drug accumulates in kidney, causing necrosis of proximal and distal renal tubules
	B. Is a dose-limiting toxicity and is cumulative with repeated doses
	C. Damage to distal renal tubules prevents reabsorption of Mg, Ca, K, with resultant decreased serum levels
	D. Peak detrimental effect usually occurs 10–20 days after treatment and is reversible
	E. Hyperuricemia may occur due to impaired tubular transport of uric acid but is responsive to allopurinol
II. *Altered nutrition, less than body requirements related to* A. Nausea and vomiting	II. A. Nausea and vomiting may be severe; begins 1 + hrs after dose, lasts 8–24 hrs, and may recur 48–72 hrs after dose
B. Taste alteration	B. Taste alterations can occur with long-term use
III. *Potential for injury related to anaphylaxis*	III. A. Anaphylactic hypersensitivity reactions have occurred (infrequently) following IV drug administration to previously treated pts

Expected Outcomes	**Nursing Interventions**
I. A. Pt will maintain normal renal function as evidenced by BUN < 20, creatinine < 1.5	I. A. Prevent nephrotoxicity with vigorous hydration and diuresis to produce urinary output of at least 100 cc/hr during treatment infusion
B. Mg, K, Ca levels will be normal	B. A typical hydration schedule is NS or D_5W 1/2 NS at 250 cc/hr for 3 hrs prior to cisplatin and for 5 hrs after; outpatient hydration would be over 1–2 hrs; diuresis is induced by the use of lasix or mannitol given prior to cisplatin administration
C. Pt will maintain baseline weight ± 5%	C. Monitor BUN and creatinine prior to initiating drug dose, as drug is excreted by the kidneys
	D. Check parameters of BUN and creatinine established in protocol
	E. Dose modifications may be made for renal impairment
	F. Concurrent use of aminoglycosides is not recommended
II. A. 1. Pt will be without nausea and vomiting 2. Nausea and vomiting, if they occur, will be minimal	II. A. 1. Premedicate with antiemetics and continue prophylactically × 24 hrs to prevent nausea and vomiting, at least for first treatment; continue antiemetic for 3–5 days after treatment ends 2. Encourage small, frequent feedings of cool, bland foods and liquids 3. Infuse cisplatin over at least 1 hr to minimize nausea and vomiting
B. Pt will eat adequate calories, proteins, minerals	B. 1. Suggest increased use of spices as tolerated 2. Help pt or significant other develop menu based on past favorite foods 3. Dietary consultation as needed
III. A. If anaphylaxis occurs, pt will maintain vital signs within normal limits	III. A. Have anaphylaxis tray with corticosteroids, antihistamines, epinephrine ready in clinic or unit where chemotherapy is administered

Cisplatin   *Continued*

Nursing Diagnosis	Defining Characteristics
III. *Potential for injury related to anaphylaxis*	B. Tachycardia, wheezing, hypotension, facial edema
	C. Usually controlled by corticosteroids, epinephrine, antihistamines
IV. *Infection and bleeding related to bone marrow depression*	IV. A. Bone marrow depression mild with low to moderate doses
	B. High-dose nadir is 2–3 weeks, with recovery in 4–5 weeks
	C. Concurrent low-dose cisplatin and radiotherapy may result in bone marrow depression
V. *Potential for activity intolerance related to anemia-induced fatigue*	V. A. Cisplatin may interfere with renal erythropoietin, causing subsequent late anemia
VI. *Potential for sensory/perceptual alterations related to neurological toxicity*	VI. A. Neurotoxicity and ototoxicity may be severe 1. Neurotoxicity: glove and stocking distribution neuropathy, with numbness, tingling, and sensory loss in arms and legs 2. Ototoxicity: high-frequency hearing loss above frequency of normal speech, affecting > 30% of pts B. 1. May be preceded by tinnitis 2. Appears dose related and can be unilateral or bilateral 3. Results from the destruction of hair cells lining organ of Corti 4. Damage is cumulative and may be permanent

Expected Outcomes	Nursing Interventions
	B. Discuss with physician the development of standing orders in case anaphylaxis occurs C. Monitor and observe pt closely during cisplatin infusions
IV. A. Pt will be without s/s of infection or bleeding	IV. A. Monitor CBC, platelet count prior to drug administration, as well as s/s infection and bleeding B. Administer growth factors (erythropoietin and GCSF) as ordered
V. A. Pt will be able to do desired activities B. Early fatigue related to anemia will resolve	V. A. Monitor hemoglobin, hematocrit B. Transfuse per MD for hematocrit < 25, s/s of severe anemia C. Teach pt about high-iron diet
VI. A. Neurotoxicity and ototoxicity will be identified early	VI. A. Assess motor and sensory function prior to therapy, and at regular intervals after each dose is given
B. If ototoxicity occurs, pt will verbalize feelings of discomfort and loss of function and identify alternative coping strategies	B. Encourage pt to verbalize feelings regarding discomfort and sensory loss

Cisplatin   *Continued*

Nursing Diagnosis	Defining Characteristics
VI. *Potential for sensory/ perceptual alterations related to neurological toxicity*	
VII. *Potential for sexual dysfunction*	VII. A. Drug is mutagenic and probably teratogenic

Expected Outcomes	Nursing Interventions
	C. Help pt discuss alternative coping strategies
	D. Baseline audiogram if high-dose platinum to be administered
	E. Repeat audiogram if pt complains of tinnitus, feeling underwater, or auditory discomfort
	F. If audiogram reveals hearing decline, discuss with pt and MD benefits/risks of further cisplatin therapy
VII. A. Pt and significant other will understand need for contraception	VII. A. As appropriate, explore with pt and significant other issues of reproductive and sexuality pattern and impact chemotherapy may have
B. Pt and significant other will identify stratgies to cope with sexual dysfunction	B. Discuss strategies to preserve sexual and reproductive health (e.g., sperm banking, contraception)

Cladribine
(Leustatin, 2-CdA)

Class: Antimetabolite

MECHANISM OF ACTION

A chlorinated purine nucleoside that selectively damages normal and
   malignant lymphocytes and monocytes that have large amounts
   of deoxycytidine kinase but small amounts of deoxynucleotidase.
   The drug enters passively through the cell membrane, is phos-
   phorylated into the active metabolite 2-CdATP, and accumulates
   in the cell. 2-CdATP interferes with DNA synthesis and prevents
   repair of DNA strand breaks in both actively dividing and normal
   cells. Process may also involve programmed cell death (apoptosis).

METABOLISM

Drug is 20% protein bound and is cleared from the plasma within 1–3
   days after cessation of treatment.

DOSAGE/RANGE

0.09 mg/kg/day IV as a continuous infusion × 7 days for one course
   of therapy (hairy cell leukemia)

DRUG PREPARATION

Available in 10-mg/10-ml preservative-free, single-use vials (1
   mg/ml), which must be further diluted in 0.9% sodium chloride
   injection. Diluted drug stable at room temperature for at least 24
   hours in normal light. Once prepared, solution may be refrigerated up to 8 hours prior to use.

Single daily dose: Add calculated drug dose to 500 ml of 0.9% sodium chloride injection, USP.

7-day continuous infusion by ambulatory infusion pump: Add calculated drug dose for 7 days to infusion reservoir using a sterile 0.22-micron hydrophilic syringe filter. Then add, again using a sterile 0.22-micron filter, sufficient sterile bacteriostatic 0.9% sodium chloride injection containing 0.9% benzyl alcohol to produce 100 ml in the infusion reservoir.

DRUG ADMINISTRATION

Administer as a continuous IV infusion for 7 days.

SPECIAL CONSIDERATIONS

Indicated for the treatment of active hairy cell leukemia, Waldenstrom's macroglobulinemia, CLL.

Unstable in 5% dextrose, so do not use D_5W as diluent.

Store unopened vials in refrigerator and protect from light.

Drug may precipitate when exposed to low temperatures. Allow solution to warm to room temperature and shake vigorously. *Do not heat or microwave.*

Drug structurally similar to pentostatin and fludarabine.

Contraindicated in patients who are hyper-sensitive to the drug.

Administer with caution in patients with renal or hepatic insufficiency.

Embryotoxic, so women of childbearing age should use contraception.

Cladribine

Nursing Diagnosis	Defining Characteristics
I. *Infection and bleeding related to bone marrow depression*	I. A. Neutropenia occurs in 70% of pts, with nadir 1–2 weeks after infusion and recovery by weeks 4–5; incidence of infection 28%, with 40% due to bacterial etiology 1. Prolonged bone marrow hypocellularity occurs in 34% of pts, lasting at least 4 months 2. Infections most common in pts with pancytopenia and lymphopenia due to hairy cell leukemia 3. Most common sites are lungs and venous access site B. Lymphopenia common, with decreased CD4 (helper T-cells) and CD8 (suppressor T-cells) and recovery by weeks 26–34 1. Incidence of infection 34% 2. Of these, 20% have viral etiology and 20% fungal etiology C. Thrombocytopenia occurs commonly, along with purpura (10%), petechia (8%), and epistaxis (5%) 1. 12–14% of pts require platelet transfusion 2. Recovery by day 12
II. *Fatigue related to anemia*	II. A. Fatigue occurs in 45% of pts B. Anemia 1. Approximately 37–44% of pts require red blood cell transfusion 2. Red cell recovery by week 8 C. Asthenia occurs in 9% of pts

Expected Outcomes	Nursing Interventions
I. A. Pt will be without s/s of infection or bleeding	I. A. Monitor Hct, WBC with differential, and platelets prior to drug administration. Discuss any abnormalities with physician
	B. Assess for s/s of infection and bleeding, and instruct pt in self-assessment and to report s/s immediately
	C. Teach pt self-care measures to minimize risk of infection and bleeding, including avoidance of OTC aspirin-containing medications
	D. Transfuse PRBCs and platelets per physician order
	E. Administer, teach self-administration of erythropoietin per physician orders
	F. Instruct pt in energy conservation and stress-reduction measures aimed at reducing fatigue
II. A. Pt will manage fatigue	II. A. Monitor hemoglobin and hematocrit and transfuse per MD order or administer erythropoietin per MD order
	B. Teach pt to alternate rest and activity
	C. Teach diet
	D. Teach stress reduction/relaxation techniques
	E. Exercise may improve energy level

Cladribine *Continued*

Nursing Diagnosis	Defining Characteristics

III. *Alteration in comfort*	III. A. Fever (> 100°F, 37.5°C) occurs in 66% of pts during the month following treatment
	  1. May be related to infection (47%)
	  2. May be related to release of endogenou pyrogen from lysed lymphocytes
	B. Other symptoms: chills (9%), diaphoresis (9%), malaise (7%), dizziness (9%), insomnia (7%), myalgia (7%), arthralgias (5%)
	C. Headache occurs in 22% of pts

IV. *Potential impairment of skin integrity*	IV. A. Rash occurs in 27–50% of pts B. Other symptoms: pruritis (6%), erythema (6%) C. Injection site reactions include erythema, swelling and pain (2%), phlebitis (2%)
V. *Alteration in nutrition*	V. A. Nausea is mild and occurs in 28% of pts B. Vomiting occurs in 13% of pts, and if antiemetics are required, it is easily controlled by phenothiazines C. Renal and hepatic function studies are rarely affected

Expected Outcomes		Nursing Interventions
III. A. Pt will be comfortable	III.	A. Assess pt for fever, chills, diaphoresis during visits; assess for s/s of infection
		B. Teach pt self-assessment, how to report this, and measures to reduce fever
		C. Anticipate laboratory and X-ray tests to rule out infection and perform according to MD order
IV. A. Pt will verbally report changes in skin and describes self-care measures	IV.	A. Assess skin for any cutaneous changes, such as rash or changes at injection site, and any associated symptoms such as pruritis; discuss with MD
		B. Instruct pt in self-care measures 1. Avoid abrasive skin products, clothing 2. Avoid tight-fitting clothing 3. Use of skin emollients appropriate for skin alteration 4. Measures to avoid scratching involved areas
		C. Consider venous access device if skin is at risk for reaction
V. A. Pt will be without nausea and vomiting	V.	A. Premedicate with antiemetics; if nausea and vomiting occur, teach pt to self-medicate with antiemetics per MD order
B. Pt will maintain weight within 5% of baseline		B. Encourage small, frequent feedings of cool, bland foods and liquids
		C. Teach pt to record diet history for 2–3 days and weekly weights
		D. If pt has decreased appetite, assess food preferences (encourage or discourage) and suggest use of spices

Cyclophosphamide
(Cytoxan, Endoxan, Endoxana, Neosar)

Class: Alkylating agent

MECHANISM OF ACTION

Causes cross-linkage in DNA strands, thus preventing DNA synthesis and cell division. Cell cycle phase-nonspecific.

METABOLISM

Inactive until converted by microsomes in liver and serum enzymes (phosphamidases). Both cyclophosphamide and its metabolites are excreted by the kidneys. Plasma half-life is 6–12 hours, with 25% of drug excreted by 8 hours. Prolonged plasma half-life in pts with renal failure results in increased myelosuppression.

DOSAGE/RANGE

400 mg/m^2 IV × 5 days
100 mg/m^2 po × 14 days
500–1500 mg/m^2 IV q 3–4 weeks

DRUG PREPARATION

Dilute vials with sterile water. Shake well. Allow solution to clear if lyophilized preparation is not used. Do not use solution unless crystals are fully dissolved. Available in 25- and 50-mg tablets.

DRUG ADMINISTRATION

PO: administer in morning or early afternoon to allow adequate excretion time. Should be taken with meals.

IV: for doses greater than 500 mg, prehydration and hemorrhagic cystitis. Administer Mesna with high-dose cyclophosphamide. Administer drug over at least 20 minutes for doses greater than 500 mg.

Solution is stable for 24 hours at room temperature, 6 days if refrigerated.

Rapid infusion may result in dizziness, nasal stuffiness, rhinorrhea, or sinus congestion during or soon after infusion.

SPECIAL CONSIDERATIONS

Metabolic and leukopenic toxicity are increased by simultaneous administration of barbiturates, corticosteroids, phenytoin, and sulfonamides.

Activity and toxicity of both cyclophosphamide and the specific drug may be altered by allopurinol, chloroquine, phenothiazines, potassium iodide, chloramphenicol, imipramine, vitamin A, warfarin, succinylcholine, digoxin, and thiazide diuretics.

Test urine for occult blood.

High-dose cyclophosphamide therapy may require catheterization and constant bladder irrigation.

Cyclophosphamide

Nursing Diagnosis	Defining Characteristics
I. *Altered nutrition, less than body requirements related to*	
A. Nausea and vomiting	I. A. Nausea and vomiting begin 2–4 hrs after dose, peak in 12 hrs, and may last 24 hrs
B. Anorexia	B. Commonly occurs
C. Stomatitis	C. Mild
D. Diarrhea	D. Infrequent and mild
E. Hepatotoxicity	E. Rare
II. *Infection and bleeding related to bone marrow depression*	II. A. Leukopenia nadir 7–14 days, with recovery in 1–2 weeks
	B. Less frequent thrombocytopenia
	C. Mild anemia

Expected Outcomes	Nursing Interventions
A. 1. Pt will be without nausea and vomiting 2. Nausea and vomiting, if they occur, will be minimal	I. A. 1. Premedicate with antiemetics and continue prophylactically × 24 hrs to prevent nausea and vomiting, at least for first treatment 2. Encourage small, frequent feedings of cool, bland foods and liquids
B. Pt will maintain baseline weight ± 5%	B. 1. Encourage small, frequent feedings of favorite foods, especially high-calorie, high-protein foods 2. Encourage use of spices 3. Weekly weights 4. Nutritional consultation as needed
C. Oral mucous membranes will remain intact and without infection	C. 1. Teach pt oral assessment 2. Encourage pt to report early stomatitis 3. Teach pt oral hygiene regimen
D. Pt will have minimal diarrhea	D. 1. Encourage pt to report onset of diarrhea 2. Administer or teach pt to self-administer antidiarrheal medications
E. Early hepatotoxicity will be identified	E. 1. Monitor LFTs (i.e., alkaline phosphatase and bilirubin) periodically during treatment 2. Monitor pt for any elevations 3. Dose modifications may be necessary if elevation occurs
II. A. Pt will be without s/s of infection or bleeding	II. A. Monitor CBC, platelet count prior to drug administration and monitor for s/s of infection and bleeding
B. Early s/s of infection or bleeding will be identified	B. Instruct pt in self-assessment of s/s of infection and bleeding C. Dose reduction often necessary (35–50%) if compromised bone marrow function

Cyclophosphamide *(continued)*

Nursing Diagnosis	Defining Characteristics
II. *Infection and bleeding related to bone marrow depression*	D. Potent immunosuppressant
III. *Potential for injury related to* A. Acute water intoxication (SIADH)	III. A. May occur with high-dose administration (> 50 mg/kg)
B. Second malignancy (bladder cancer, acute leukemia)	B. Prolonged therapy may cause bladder cancer (related to local toxicity of drug metabolites) and acute leukemia (related to prolonged bone marrow toxicity)
IV. *Altered urinary elimination related to hemorrhagic cystitis*	IV. A. Metabolites of cyclophosphamide, if allowed to accumulate in bladder, irritate bladder wall capillaries, causing hemorrhagic cystitis B. Sterile chemical cystitis occurs in 5–10% of pts C. Evidenced by hematuria, gross or microscopic (> 20 RBC) D. Mesna frequently used to avoid hemorrhagic cystitis E. Can also cause bladder fibrosis
V. *Alteration in cardiac output related to high-dose cyclophosphamide*	V. A. Cardiomyopathy may occur with high doses; also, potentiates cardiotoxicity of doxorubicin (Adriamycin)

Expected Outcomes	Nursing Interventions
	D. Administration of GCSF often necessary with high-dose therapy
III. A. SIADH will be identified early	III. A. 1. If high-dose cytoxan administered, monitor serum sodium, osmolality, and urine electrolytes and osmolality 2. Strictly monitor I&O and total body balance 3. Daily weights 4. Water restrictions as ordered
B. Malignancy, if it occurs, will be identified early	B. Pts receiving prolonged therapy should be screened
IV. A. Pt will be without hemorrhagic cystitis	IV. A. Monitor BUN and creatinine prior to drug dose, as drug is excreted by kidneys B. Provide or instruct pt in hydration of at least 3 liters of fluid/day C. Encourage voiding to empty bladder at least q 2–3 hours and at bedtime D. Assess pt for s/s and instruct pt to report hematuria, urinary frequency, dysuria E. Instruct pt that oral cyclophosphamide should be taken early in day to prevent accumulation of drug in the bladder F. Administer Mesna as ordered
V. A. Early s/s of cardiomyopathy will be identified	V. A. If pt is receiving high-dose cyclophosphamide, assess for s/s of cardiomyopathy B. Gated blood pool scan (GBPS) or echocardiogram often used to check LVEF (left ventricular ejection fraction) C. Assess quality and regularity of heartbeat

Cyclophosphamide   *Continued*

Nursing Diagnosis	Defining Characteristics
V. *Alteration in cardiac output related to high-dose cyclophosphamide*	
VI. *Potential for impaired gas exchange related to pulmonary toxicity*	VI. A. Rare, but may occur with prolonged, high-dose therapy or continuous low-dose therapy B. Appears as interstitial pneumonitis and onset insidious C. May respond to steroids
VII. *Altered body image related to* A. Alopecia B. Changes in nails, skin	VII. A. 1. Occurs in 30–50% of pts, especially with IV dosing 2. Some degree of hair loss expected in all pts 3. Begins after 3+ weeks and may grow back while on therapy 4. May be slight to diffuse thinning B. Hyperpigmentation of nails and skin, transverse ridging of nails ("banding") may occur
VIII. *Sexual dysfunction*	VIII. A. Drug is mutagenic and teratogenic B. Testicular atrophy sometimes occurs with reversible oligo- and azoospermia C. Amenorrhea often occurs in females D. Drug is excreted in breast milk

Expected Outcomes	**Nursing Interventions**
	D. Instruct pt to report dyspnea, shortness of breath
VI. A. Early s/s of pulmonary toxicity will be identified	VI. A. If pt is receiving high-dose or continuous low-dose cyclophosphamide, assess for s/s of pulmonary dysfunction B. Discuss pulmonary function studies to be performed periodically with MD C. Assess lung sounds prior to drug administration D. Instruct pt to report cough or dyspnea
VII. A. Pt will verbalize feelings re hair loss and identify strategies to cope with change in body image	VII. A. 1. Assess pt for s/s of hair loss 2. Discuss with pt impact of hair loss and strategies to minimize distress (i.e., wig, scarf, cap) 3. Begin discussion before therapy has been initiated
B. Pt will verbalize feelings re changes in nail or skin color or texture and identify strategies to cope with change in body image	B. 1. Assess pt for changes in skin, nails 2. Discuss with pt impact of of changes and strategies to minimize distress (i.e., wearing nail polish, long sleeves)
VIII. A. Pt and significant other will understand need for contraception	VIII. A. As appropriate, explore with pt and significant other issues of reproductive and sexuality pattern and the impact chemotherapy will have
B. Pt and significant other will identify strategies to cope with sexual dysfunction	B. Discuss strategies to preserve sexual and reproductive health (e.g., sperm banking, contraception)

Cytarabine, cytosine arabinoside
(Ara-C, Cytosar-U, Arabinosyl Cytosine)

Class: Antimetabolite

MECHANISM OF ACTION

Antimetabolite (pyrimidine analogue) that is incorporated into DNA, slowing its synthesis and causing defects in the linkages in new DNA fragments. Also, cells exposed to cytarabine in the S phase reinitiate DNA synthesis when the drug is removed, resulting in erroneous duplication of the early portions of the DNA strands. Most effective when cells are undergoing rapid DNA synthesis.

METABOLISM

Inactivated by liver enzymes in biphasic manner: half-lives 10–15 minutes and 2–3 hours. Crosses the blood-brain barrier with CSF concentration of 50% that of plasma; 70% of dose excreted in urine as Ara-U; 4–10% excreted 12–24 hours after administration.

DOSAGE/RANGE

Leukemia: 100 mg/m^2 day IV continuous infusion × 5–10 days
100 mg/m^2 every 12 hours × 1–3 weeks IV or SQ
Head and neck: 1 mg/kg every 12 hours × 5–7 days IV or SQ
High dose: 2–3 mg/m^2 IV
Differentiation: 10 mg/m^2 SQ every 12 hours × 15–21 days
Intrathecal: 20–30 mg/m^2

DRUG PREPARATION

100-mg vials: Add water with benzyl alcohol, then dilute with NS or
  D_5W.

500-mg vials: Add water with benzyl alcohol, then dilute with NS or
  D_5W.

For intrathecal use and high dose: Use preservative-free diluent.

Reconstituted drug is stable 48 hours at room temperature and 7 days
  refrigerated.

DRUG ADMINISTRATION

Doses of 100–200 mg can be given SQ.

Doses less than 1 gm: Administer via volutrol over 10–20 minutes.

Doses over 1 gm: Administer over 2 hours.

SPECIAL CONSIDERATIONS

Thrombophlebitis or pain at the injection site should be treated with
  warm compresses.

Dizziness has occurred with too-rapid IV infusions.

Use with caution if hepatic dysfunction exists.

May decrease bioavailability of digoxin when given in combination.

Cytarabine, cytosine arabinoside

Nursing Diagnosis	Defining Characteristics
I. *Altered nutrition, less than body requirements related to* A. Nausea and vomiting	I. A. 1. Occurs in 50% of pts 2. Dose related 3. Lasts for several hours
B. Anorexia	B. Commonly occurs
C. Stomatitis	C. Occurs 7–10 days after therapy is initiated in about 15% of pts
D. Diarrhea	D. Infrequent and mild
E. Hepatotoxicity	E. Usually mild and reversible, but drug should be used cautiously in pts with hepatic dysfunction
II. *Infection and bleeding related to bone marrow depression*	II. A. Related to dose and duration of therapy B. Leukopenic nadir 7–14 days after drug administration; recovery in 3 weeks C. Thrombocytopenia common

Expected Outcomes	Nursing Interventions
I. A. 1. Pt will be without nausea or vomiting 2. Nausea and vomiting, if they occur, will be minimal	I. A. 1. Premedicate with antiemetics and continue prophylactically × 24 hrs to prevent nausea and vomiting, at least for first treatment 2. Encourage small, frequent feedings of cool, bland foods and liquids 3. I&O, daily weights if inpatient (assess for s/s of fluid and electrolyte imbalance)
B. Pt will maintain baseline weight ± 5%	B. 1. Encourage small, frequent feedings of favorite foods, especially high-calorie, high-protein foods 2. Encourage use of spices 3. Weekly weights, daily if inpatient
C. Oral mucous membranes will remain intact and without signs of infection	C. 1. Assess oral cavity every day: teach pt to do own oral assessment and oral hygiene regimen 2. Encourage pt to report early stomatitis 3. Pain relief measures, if indicated
D. Pt will have minimal diarrhea	D. 1. Encourage pt to report onset of diarrhea 2. Administer or teach pt to administer antidiarrheal medication
E. Early hepatotoxicity will be identified	E. 1. Monitor LFTs prior to drug dose, especially with high drug doses 2. Assess pt prior to and during treatment for s/s hepatotoxicity
II. A. Pt will be without s/s of infection or bleeding	II. A. Monitor CBC, platelet count prior to drug administration, as well as s/s of infection and bleeding
B. Early s/s of bleeding and infection will be identified	B. Assess pt q day for s/s of infection and bleeding; instruct pt in self-assessment C. Transfuse as necessary with red cells, platelets

Cytarabine, cytosine arabinoside *Continued*

Nursing Diagnosis	Defining Characteristics
II. *Infection and bleeding related to bone marrow depression*	D. Megaloblastic changes in the marrow are common E. Anemia seen frequently F. Potent but transient suppression of primary and secondary antibody responses
III. *Impaired skin integrity related to alopecia*	III. A. Occurs frequently
IV. *Potential for injury related to* A. Neurotoxicity	IV. A. 1. Can occur with high doses 2. Cerebellar toxicity is indication for immediate cessation for therapy 3. Lethargy, somnolence have resulted from too-rapid infusions of drug
B. Tumor lysis syndrome (TLS), hyperuricemia	B. 1. TLS may develop secondary to rapid lysis of tumor cells 2. Usually begins 1–5 days after initiation of chemotherapy

Expected Outcomes	Nursing Interventions
	D. Administer growth factors (erythropoietin & GCSF) as ordered
	III. A. Pt will verbalize feelings re hair loss and identify strategies to cope with change in body image B. Discuss with pt impact of hair loss and strategies to minimize distress (i.e., wig, scarf, cap); begin before therapy is initiated
IV. A. 1. Early cerebellar toxicity will be recognized and reported 2. Neurotoxicity will be minimized	IV. A. 1. Assess pt q shift and before administering drug for cerebellar toxicity 2. Instruct pt in self-assessment of cerebellar function; encourage pt to report changes in coordination, control of eye movement, etc. 3. Report changes in cerebellar function 4. Administer drug according to established guidelines; monitor pt during infusion for lethargy, somnolence
B. Serum uric acid, potassium, and phosphorus will remain within normal limits	B. 1. Monitor BUN, creatinine, potassium, phosphorus, uric acid, and calcium 2. Monitor I&O 3. Monitor for renal, cardiac, neuromuscular s/s of TLS 4. Administer allopurinol, fluids as ordered

Cytarabine liposome injection
(DepoCyt)

Class: Antimetabolite

MECHANISM OF ACTION

Drug is converted to the metabolite ara-CTP intracellularly. Ara-CTP is thought to inhibit DNA polymerase, thereby affecting DNA synthesis. Incorporation into DNA and RNA may also contribute to cytarabine cellular toxicity.

METABOLISM

With systemically administered cytarabine, the drug is metabolized to an inactive compound, ara-U, and is then renally excreted. In the CSF, however, conversion to the ara-U is negligible, because CNS tissue and CSF lack the enzyme necessary for the conversion to occur.

DOSAGE/RANGE

Indicated for the intrathecal treatment of lymphomatous meningitis only. To be given as follows:

Induction therapy: DepoCyt, 50 mg, administered intrathecally (intraventricular or lumbar puncture) every 14 days for 2 doses (weeks 1 and 3).

Consolidation therapy: DepoCyt, 50 mg, administered intrathecally (intraventricular or lumbar puncture) every 14 days for 3 doses (weeks 5, 7, and 9) followed by 1 additional dose at week 13.

Maintenance therapy: DepoCyt, 50 mg, administered intrathecally
(intraventricular or lumbar puncture) every 28 days for 4 doses
(weeks 17, 21, 25, and 29).

If drug-related neurotoxicity develops, the dose should be reduced
to 25 mg. If toxicity persists, treatment with DepoCyt should be
terminated.

DRUG PREPARATION/ADMINISTRATION

Drug is supplied in single-use vials and comes as a white to off-white
suspension in 5 ml of fluid.

Drug is to be withdrawn immediately before use and should not be
used later than 4 hours from the time of withdrawal from vial.

DepoCyt should be administered directly into the CSF over 1–5 minutes. Pts should lie flat for 1 hour after administration.

Pts should be started on dexamethasone 4 mg bid either PO or IV for
5 days beginning on the day of DepoCyt injection.

SPECIAL CONSIDERATIONS

Do not use inline filters with DepoCyt: administer directly into CSF.

Must be administered with concurrent dexa-methasone as described
above.

Cytarabine liposome injection

Nursing Diagnosis	Defining Characteristics
I. *Alteration in nutrition, less than body requirements, related to nausea and vomiting*	I. A. Nausea, vomiting, and headache are common, and are physical manifestations of chemical arachnoiditis
II. *Alteration in comfort related to headache, neck and/or back pain, fever*	II. A. Some degree of chemical arachnoiditis is expected in about a third of pts: incidence approaches 100% of pts; when dexamethasone is *not* given with DepoCyt B. Causes headache, neck pain and/or rigidity, back pain, fever

Expected Outcomes		Nursing Interventions	
I.	A. Nausea/vomiting will be avoided or minimized	I.	A. Administer dexamethasone throughout treatment course as described above B. Observe pt for at least 1 hr after administration for toxicity C. Administer antiemetics as ordered. Teach pt to report nausea/vomiting and to self-administer antiemetics D. Encourage small, frequent feedings of cool, bland foods
II.	A. Pt will report comfort throughout treatment course B. Discomfort will be identified early and treated effectively	II.	A. Instruct pt in dexamethasone self-administration and to report to MD if oral doses are not tolerated B. Pts should lie flat for 1 hr after lumbar puncture and should be observed for immediate toxic reactions C. Administer medications to treat pain

Dacarbazine
(DTIC-Dome, Imidazole carboximide)

Class: Alkylating agent

MECHANISM OF ACTION

Unclear, but appears to be an agent that methylates nucleic acids (particularly DNA), causing cross-linkage and breaks in DNA strands. This inhibits RNA and DNA synthesis. Also interacts with sulfhydryl groups in proteins. Generally, cell cycle phase-nonspecific.

METABOLISM

Thought to be activated by liver microsomes. Excreted renally, with a plasma half-life of 0.65 hour, and terminal half-life of 5 hours.

DOSAGE/RANGE

375 mg/m^2 every 3–4 weeks

> *or*

150–250 mg/m^2 day × 5 days, repeat every 3–4 weeks

> *or*

800–900 mg/m^2 as a single dose every 3–4 weeks

DRUG PREPARATION

Add sterile water or NS to vial.

DRUG ADMINISTRATION

Administer via volutrol over 20 minutes or give via IV push over 2–3 minutes.

Stable for 8 hours at room temperature, 72 hours if refrigerated. Store lyophilized drug in refrigerator and protect from light. Drug decomposition is denoted by a change in color from yellow to pink.

SPECIAL CONSIDERATIONS

Irritant—avoid extravasation.

Pain may occur above site. Usually unrelieved by slowing IV, but may be relieved by applying ice to painful area. May cause venospasm; slow rate if this occurs.

Anaphylaxis has occurred with infusion of dacarbazine.

Drug interactions: increased drug metabolism with concurrent administration of dilantin, phenobarbital; potential increased toxicity with Imuran and 6-MP.

Dacarbazine

Nursing Diagnosis	Defining Characteristics

I. *Altered nutrition, less than body requirements related to*
   A. Nausea and vomiting
	I.
	  A. 90% incidence of nausea and vomiting, moderate to severe, beginning 1–3 hrs after dose; tolerance develops when given over several days, so nausea and vomiting are less severe

B. Diarrhea	B. Uncommon
C. Anorexia	C. Commonly occurs; may also cause metallic taste sensation
D. Hepatotoxicity	D. Rare; however, hepatic veno-occlusive disease has been described (hepatic vein thrombosis and hepatocellular necrosis)

II. *Infection and bleeding related to bone marrow depression*	II.
	  A. Nadir 14–28 days following treatment
	
	  B. Anemia may occur with long-term treatment

III. *Potential for injury related to anaphylaxis*	III. A. Anaphylaxis may occur rarely, with fever, confusion, urticaria, wheezing, or hypotension

Expected Outcomes	**Nursing Interventions**

I. A. 1. Pt will be without nausea and vomiting
     2. Nausea and vomiting, if they occur, will be minimal
	I. A. 1. Premedicate with antiemetic
	     2. Help pt relax using distraction, progressive muscle relaxation, imagery; teach pt how to induce relaxation
	     3. Infuse drug slowly over 1 hr to decrease nausea and vomiting

B. Diarrhea, if it occurs, will abate	B. 1. Assess pt for evidence of diarrhea 2. Administer antidiarrheal medication or teach pt to self-administer

C. Pt will maintain baseline weight ± 5%	C. 1. Encourage small, frequent feedings of favorite foods, especially high-calorie, high-protein foods
	    2. Encourage use of spices
	    3. Weekly weight

D. Hepatocellular dysfunction, if it occurs, will be identified early	D. 1. Monitor LFTs prior to treatment 2. If LFTs are elevated, discuss withholding medication with MD
II. A. Pt will be without s/s of infection or bleeding	II. A. Monitor CBC, platelet count prior to drug administration, as well as s/s of infection and bleeding
B. Early s/s of infection or bleeding will be identified	B. Instruct pt in self-assessment of s/s of infection and bleeding C. Transfuse with red cells, platelets per MD order
III. A. Allergic reaction or anaphylaxis, if it occurs, will be detected early	III. A. Review standing orders for management of pt in anaphylaxis and identify location of anaphylaxis kit containing epinephrine 1:1000, hydrocortisone sodium succinate (Solucortef), diphenhydramine HCl (Benadryl), Aminophylline, and others
B. Airway will remain patent C. BP will remain within 20 mmHg of baseline	B. Prior to drug administration, obtain baseline vital signs and record mental status

Dacarbazine   *Continued*

Nursing Diagnosis	Defining Characteristics
III. *Potential for injury related to anaphylaxis*	

Expected Outcomes	Nursing Interventions
	C. Observe for following s/s during infusion, usually occurring within first 15 mins of start of infusion
	D. Future allergic responses will be prevented
	1. *Subjective*
	a. Generalized itching
	b. Chest tightness
	c. Difficulty speaking
	d. Agitation
	e. Uneasiness
	f. Dizziness
	g. Nausea
	h. Crampy abdominal pain
	i. Anxiety
	j. Sense of impending doom
	k. Desire to urinate/defecate
	l. Chills
	2. *Objective*
	a. Flushed appearance (angioedema of face, neck, eyelids, hands, feet)
	b. Localized or generalized urticaria
	c. Respiratory distress ± wheezing
	d. Hypotension
	e. Cyanosis
	E. If reaction occurs, stop infusion and notify MD
	F. Place pt in supine position to promote perfusion of visceral organs
	G. Monitor vital signs until stable
	H. Provide emotional reassurance to pt and family
	I. Maintain patent airway and have ready equipment for CPR if needed
	J. Document incident
	K. Discuss with MD desensitization versus drug discontinuance for further dosing

Dacarbazine *Continued*

Nursing Diagnosis	Defining Characteristics

IV. *Alteration in comfort related to*
  A. "Flu-like syndrome"
	IV. A. 1. Influenza-like syndrome characterized by malaise, headache, myalgia, chills, and hypotension
	     2. May occur up to 7 days after first dose, last 7–21 days, and recur with subsequent doses

B. Pain at injection site	B. Drug is an *irritant* and may cause phlebitis of vein
V. *Impaired skin integrity related to* A. Alopecia	V. A. Causes alopecia in 90% of pts, with obvious impact on body image

Expected Outcomes	**Nursing Interventions**
IV. A. Pt will verbalize increased comfort	IV. A. 1. Discuss possibility of flu-like syndrome occurring 2. Suggest symptom management with acetaminophen as needed 3. Encourage fluids orally ≥ 3 L/day, rest 4. Encourage pt to verbalize feelings and give other emotional support

B. Pain will be minimized	B. 1. Assess pt for appropriateness of central venous access device, especially if pt will receive successive treatments
	2. Administer DTIC in 100–250 cc IV fluid and infuse slowly over 1 hr
	3. Consider premedication and discuss with MD:
	   a. Apply ice or heat above injection site to reduce venous burning
	   b. Premedicate with hydrocortisone IVP, lidocaine 1–2% IVP, or heparin IVP to minimize trauma to vein prior to DTIC infusion (DTIC forms precipitate with hydrocortisone sodium succinate [Solucortef] but not with hydrocortisone)

V. A. Pt will verbalize expected side effects relating to hair loss and strategies to minimize distress related to these side effects	V. A. 1. Encourage pt to obtain wig prior to hair loss 2. Encourage pt to verbalize feelings re anticipated or actual hair loss and discuss strategies to minimize impact of alopecia 3. Provide emotional support

Dacarbazine   *Continued*

Nursing Diagnosis	Defining Characteristics
B. Facial flushing, erythema, and urticaria	B. Facial flushing occurs rarely and is self-limiting; erythema and urticaria are rare but may occur around injection site
VI. *Potential for sensory/ perceptual alterations*	VI. A. Facial paresthesia, photosensitivity
VII. *Potential for sexual dysfunction*	VII. A. Drug is teratogenic

Expected Outcomes	Nursing Interventions
B. Pt will verbalize feelings re changes in skin and identify strategies to cope with these changes	B. 1. Assess pt for changes in skin 2. Discuss with pt impact of changes and strategies to minimize distress
VI. A. Pt will verbalize expected side effects and self-care measures	VI. A. Instruct pt in self-care measures if sensory changes occur 1. To report facial paresthesias to nurse 2. To avoid strong sunlight, wear sunscreen on skin and protective clothing and hat
VII. A. Pt and significant other will verbalize importance of and need for contraception	VII. A. As appropriate, discuss birth control measures 1. Discuss reproductive goals, hopes, and impact contraception will have 2. Provide teaching booklets

Dactinomycin
(Actinomycin D, Cosmegan)

Class: Antitumor antibiotic isolated from *streptomyces* fungus

MECHANISM OF ACTION

Binds to guanine portion of DNA and blocks the ability of DNA to act
as a template for both DNA and RNA. At lower drug doses, the
predominant action inhibits RNA, whereas at higher doses both
RNA and DNA are inhibited. Cell cycle-specific for G_1 and S
phases.

METABOLISM

Most of drug is excreted unchanged in bile and urine. There is a rapid
clearance of drug from plasma (approximately 36 hours). Dose reduction in the presence of liver or renal failure may be needed.

DOSAGE/RANGE

10–15 μg/kg/day × 5 days every 3–4 weeks
15–30 μg/kg/week, 400–600 μg/m^2 day for 5 days IV
Frequency and schedule may vary according to protocol and age.

DRUG PREPARATION

Add sterile water for a concentration of 500 μg/ml. Use preservative-
free water, as precipitate may develop otherwise.

DRUG ADMINISTRATION

Usually given IV push via sidearm of running IV.

SPECIAL CONSIDERATIONS

Drug is a vesicant. Give through a running IV to avoid extravasation,
which may develop into ulceration, necrosis, and pain.

Skin changes—radiation recall phenomenon. Skin discoloration along
vein used for injection.

Dactinomycin

Nursing Diagnosis	Defining Characteristics
I. *Potential for infection and bleeding related to bone marrow depression*	I. A. Onset 7–10 days, nadir 14–21 days, with recovery 21–28 days B. Anemia is delayed C. Myelosuppression may be dose limiting and severe
II. *Alteration in nutrition* A. Nausea and vomiting	II. A. Beginning 2–5 hrs after dose, may last 24 hrs
B. Diarrhea, cramps	B. 30% incidence
C. Anorexia	C. Occurs frequently
III. *Alteration in mucous membranes, including stomatitis, esophagitis, proctitus*	III. A. There is an incidence of irritation of mucous membranes lining the entire gastrointestinal tract

Expected Outcomes	Nursing Interventions
I. A. Pt will be without infection or bleeding B. Early s/s of infection and bleeding will be identified	I. A. Monitor CBC, platelet count prior to drug administration B. Assess pt and teach pt self-assessment for s/s of infection and bleeding C. Transfuse red cells, platelets per MD order D. Drug dosage should be reduced for lower than normal blood values E. Administer growth factors as ordered
II. A. 1. Pt will be without nausea and vomiting 2. Nausea and vomiting, if they occur, will be minimal B. Pt will have minimal diarrhea C. Pt will maintain baseline weight ± 5%	II. A. 1. Premedicate with antiemetics and continue prophylactically × 24 hrs to prevent nausea and vomiting, at least first treatment 2. Encourage small, frequent feedings of cool, bland foods and liquids 3. Administer oral dose on an empty stomach B. 1. Encourage pt to report onset of diarrhea 2. Administer or teach pt to self-administer antidiarrheal medication C. 1. Encourage small, frequent feedings of favorite foods, especially high-calorie, high-protein foods 2. Encourage use of spices 3. Weekly weights
III. A. 1. Oral mucous membranes will remain intact and without infection 2. The gastrointestinal toxicity will be minimal	III. A. Teach pt oral assessment and oral hygiene regimen B. Encourage pt to report early stomatitis C. Teach pt importance of stomatitis and the entire gastrointestinal system D. Administer pain medications/topical anesthetics as needed E. Guaiac all stools

Dactinomycin *Continued*

Nursing Diagnosis	Defining Characteristics
IV. *Impaired skin integrity*	IV. A. Radiation recall at previously irradiated skin site
	B. Acne-like rash and alopecia can occur in 47% of pts
	C. Drug is a vesicant

Expected Outcomes	Nursing Interventions
IV. A. Pt will verbalize feelings re changes in nail or skin color, texture	IV. A. 1. Assess pt for changes in skin, nails, and hair loss 2. Discuss with pt impact of changes and strategies to minimize distress
B. Identify strategies to cope with change in body image	B. 1. Discuss skin changes as they relate to changes in body image

C. Extravasation, if it occurs, will be detected early with early intervention	C. 1. Use careful technique during venipuncture
	2. Administer vesicant through freely flowing IV, constantly monitoring IV site and pt response
	3. Nurse should be *thoroughly* familiar with institutional policy and procedure for administration of a vesicant agent
	4. If vesicant drug is administered as a continuous infusion, drug must be given through a patent central line
	5. If extravasation is suspected:
	    a. Stop drug being administered
	    b. Aspirate any residual drug and blood from IV tubing, IV catheter/needle, and IV site if possible
	    c. If antidote exists, instill antidote into area of apparent infiltration as per MD orders and institutional policy and procedure
	    d. Apply cold or topical medication as per MD order and institutional policy and procedure
	6. Assess site regularly for pain, progression of erythema, induration, and evidence of necrosis

D. Skin and underlying tissue damage will be minimized	

Dactinomycin *Continued*

Nursing Diagnosis	Defining Characteristics
IV. *Impaired skin integrity*	
V. *Alteration in comfort*	V. A. Flu-like symptoms may occur, including malaise, myalgia, fever, depression
VI. *Alteration in metabolism* A. Hepatotoxicity B. Renal toxicity	VI. A. Drug is metabolized rapidly by the liver B. Drug is metabolized rapidly by the kidney
VII. *Potential for sexual dysfunction*	VII. A. Drug is mutagenic and teratogenic

Expected Outcomes	Nursing Interventions
	7. When in doubt about whether drug is infiltrating, *treat as infiltration*
	8. Teach pt to assess site and notify MD if condition worsens
	9. Arrange next clinic visit for assessment of site depending on drug, amount infiltrated, extent of potential injury, and pt variables
	10. Document in pt record as per institutional policy and procedure
V. A. Pt will remain comfortable during therapy	V. A. Assess pt for symptoms during and after treatment B. Premedicate with acetaminophen, antihistamine, or steroids as per MD order C. Evaluate the effectiveness of the symptomatic relief that is prescribed and administered
VI. A. Hepatic dysfunction will be identified early B. Renal toxicity will be minimal	VI. A. 1. Establish a baseline for liver function tests 2. Monitor SGOT, SGPT, LDH, alkaline phosphatase, and bilirubin on a regular basis 3. Notify MD of any elevations B. 1. Monitor BUN and creatinine prior to drug dose 2. Provide fluid and teach pt the importance of hydration
VII. A. Pt and significant other will understand need for contraception B. Pt and significant other will identify strategies to cope with sexual dysfunction	VII. A. As appropriate, explore with pt and significant other reproductive patterns and impact chemotherapy will have B. Discuss strategies to preserve sexuality and reproductive health (sperm banking, contraception)

Daunorubicin hydrochloride
(Cerubidine, Daunomycin)

Class: Anthracycline antibiotic isolated from streptomycin products, in particular the rhodomycin products

MECHANISM OF ACTION

No clearly defined mechanism. Intercalates DNA, therefore blocking DNA, RNA, and protein synthesis. Binds to DNA and inhibits DNA replication and DNA-dependent RNA synthesis.

METABOLISM

Site of significant metabolism is in the liver. Doses need to be modified in presence of abnormal liver function. Excreted in urine and bile.

DOSAGE/RANGE

30–60 mg/m^2/day IV for 3 consecutive days

DRUG PREPARATION

Add sterile water to produce liquid. Drug will form a precipitate when mixed with heparin and is incompatible with dexamethasone.

DRUG ADMINISTRATION

Give IV push through the sidearm of a freely flowing IV or as a bolus over 1–2 hours or as a continuous infusion over 24 hours. Must be given via a central line if given via bolus or continuous infusion, as drug is a potent vesicant.

SPECIAL CONSIDERATIONS

Drug is a potent vesicant. Give through running IV to avoid extravasation.

Moderate to severe nausea and vomiting occur in 50% of patients within first 24 hours.

Causes discoloration of urine (pink to red for up to 48 hours after administration).

Cardiac toxicity—dose limit at 550 mg/m^2. Patients may exhibit irreversible congestive heart failure. Acute toxicity may be seen within hours after administration. This is unrelated to cumulative dose and may manifest symptoms of pump or conduction function. Rarely, transient EKG abnormalities, CHF, pericardial effusion (whole syndrome referred to as myocarditis-pericarditis syndrome) may occur, which may lead to demise of patient.

Daunorubicin hydrochloride

Nursing Diagnosis	Defining Characteristics
I. *Potential for infection and bleeding related to bone marrow depression*	I. A. Leukopenia onset in 7 days; nadir 10–14 days; recovery 21–28 days B. Thrombocytopenia occurs with BMD
II. *Potential for altered cardiac output*	II. A. Acute: 6–30% of pts develop transient EKG changes 1–3 days after dose B. Chronic: cumulative, dose-related cardiomyopathy C. CHF may develop 1–16 months after therapy ceases
III. *Alteration in nutrition, less than body requirements*	III. A. Mild nausea, vomiting day of therapy (50% incidence) B. Infrequent stomatitis 3–7 days after dose

Expected Outcomes	Nursing Interventions

I.   A. Pt will be without s/s of infection or bleeding
    B. Early s/s of infection and bleeding will be identified
	I. A. Monitor CBC, platelet count prior to drug administration
	    B. Monitor s/s of infection and bleeding
	    C. Instruct pt in self-assessment of s/s of infection and bleeding
	    D. Dose reduction may be necessary
	    E. Transfuse with red cells, platelets per MD order
	    F. Administer growth factors as ordered

II. A. Early s/s of cardiomyopathy will be identified	II. A. Assess for s/s of cardiomyopathy
	    B. Assess quality and regularity of heartbeat
	    C. Baseline EKG
	    D. Instruct pt to report dyspnea, shortness of breath, swelling of extremities, orthopnea
	    E. Chronic cardiomyopathy: monitor gated blood pool scan (GBPS) and ejection fraction, baseline and periodically through treatment as cumulative dosages approach maximum

III. A. Pt will be without nausea and vomiting, or if they occur, will be minimal
 	
    B. Oral mucous membranes will remain intact
	III. A. 1. Premedicate with antiemetic, as ordered, and continue prophylactically to prevent nausea and vomiting
	       2. Encourage small, frequent feedings of cool, bland foods and liquids
	    B. 1. Encourage small, frequent feedings of favorite foods, especially high-calorie, high-protein foods
	       2. Encourage use of spices
	       3. Weekly weights
	       4. Assess oral mucous membranes
	       5. Instruct pt in oral assessment and mouth care

Daunorubicin hydrochloride *Continued*

Nursing Diagnosis	Defining Characteristics
IV. *Potential for impaired skin integrity* A. Extravasation	IV. A. Extravasation of drug can cause tissue necrosis
B. Alopecia	B. Alopecia (complete) 3–4 weeks after treatment begins
C. Skin reactions	C. Reactivation of radiation induced lesions (radiation recall); hyperpigmentation, rash; onycholysis (nail loosening from nail bed)

Expected Outcomes	**Nursing Interventions**

IV. A. Extravasation, if it occurs, is detected early, with early intervention; skin and underlying tissue damage is minimized	IV. A. 1. Use careful technique during venipuncture
	2. Administer vesicant through freely flowing IV, constantly monitoring IV site and pt response
	3. Nurse should be thoroughly familiar with institutional policy and procedure for administration of a vesicant agent
	4. If vesicant drug is administered as a continuous infusion, drug must be given through a patent central line
	5. If extravasation is suspected:
	  a. Stop drug being administered
	  b. Aspirate any residual drug and blood from IV tubing, IV catheter/needle, and IV site if possible
	  c. *If antidote exists,* instill antidote into area of apparent infiltration as per MD orders and institutional policy and procedure
	  d. Apply cold or topical medication as per MD order and institutional policy and procedure
	6. Assess site regularly for pain, progression of erythema, induration, and evidence of necrosis
	7. When in doubt whether drug is infiltrating, *treat as an infiltration*
	8. Teach pt to assess site and notify MD if condition worsens

Daunorubicin hydrochloride   *Continued*

Nursing Diagnosis	**Defining Characteristics**
B. Alopecia	B. Alopecia (complete) 3–4 weeks after treatment begins
C. Skin reactions	C. Reactivation of radiation induced lesions (radiation recall); hyperpigmentation, rash; onycholysis (nail loosening from nail bed)
V. *Potential for sexual dysfunction*	V. A. Drug is mutagenic and teratogenic
VI. *Potential for alteration in comfort, i.e., pain*	VI. A. Abdominal pain may occur

Expected Outcomes		**Nursing Interventions**	
			9. Arrange next clinic visit for assessment of site depending on drug, amount infiltrated, extent of potential injury, and pt variables
			10. Document in pt record as per institutional policy and procedure
	B. Pt will verbalize feelings re hair loss and identify strategies to cope with changes in body images	B.	1. Discuss with pt impact of hair loss
			2. Suggest wig as appropriate prior to actual hair loss
			3. Explore with pt response to actual hair loss and plan strategies to minimize distress (e.g., wig, scarf, cap)
	C. Skin discomfort will be minimized and skin will remain intact; pt will verbalize feelings re skin changes	C.	1. This is not an indication to stop the drug
			2. Discuss with MD symptomatic management
			3. Reinforce pt teaching on the action and side effects of daunorubicin
			4. Offer emotional support
V.	A. Pt and significant other will understand the need for contraception	V.	A. As appropriate, explore with pt and significant other reproductive and sexuality pattern and impact chemotherapy will have
	B. Pt and significant other will identify strategies to cope with sexual dysfunction		B. Discuss strategies to preserve sexuality and reproductive health (e.g., sperm banking, contraception)
VI.	A. Pt will be supported during therapy	VI.	A. Offer emotional support to pt
			B. Reinforce information on the action and side effects of daunorubicin hydrochloride
			C. Discuss with MD medicating for the pain

Daunorubicin citrate liposome injection
(DaunoXome)

Class: Anthracycline antibiotic that is isolated from streptomycin products, in particular the rhodomycin products, and encapsulated in a liposome

MECHANISM OF ACTION

No clearly defined mechanism. Intercalates DNA, therefore blocking DNA, RNA, and protein synthesis. Binds to DNA and inhibits DNA replication and DNA-dependent RNA synthesis. Drug is encapsulated within liposomes (lipid vesicles) and is preferentially delivered to solid tumor sites. The liposomal encapsulated drug is protected from chemical and enzymatic degradation, protein binding, and uptake by normal tissues while circulating in the blood. The exact mechanism for selective targeting of tumor sites is unknown but is believed to be related to increased permeability of the tumor neovasculature. Once delivered to the tumor, the drug is slowly released and exerts its antineoplastic action.

METABOLISM

Cleared from the plasma at 17 ml/min with a small steady-state volume of distribution. As compared to standard IV daunorubicin, the liposomal encapsulated daunorubicin has higher daunorubicin exposure (plasma area under the curve, ARC). The elimination half-life (4.4 hours) is shorter than standard daunorubicin.

DOSAGE/RANGE

$40 \text{ mg/m}^2/\text{day}$ IV bolus over 60 minutes every 2 weeks

DRUG PREPARATION

Drug is available as 50 mg of daunorubicin base in a total volume of 25 ml (2 mg/ml).

Visually inspect for particulate matter and discoloration (drug appears as a translucent dispersion of liposomes that scatters light but should not be opaque or have precipitate or foreign matter present).

Withdraw the calculated volume of drug and add to an equal volume of 5% dextrose to deliver a 1:1, or 1 mg/ml solution.

Administer immediately, or may be stored in the refrigerator at 2–8°C (36–46°F) for 6 hours.

Use ONLY 5% dextrose, NOT 0.9% sodium chloride or any other solution.

Drug contains no preservatives.

Unopened drug vials should be stored in the refrigerator at 2–8°C (36–46°F), but should not be frozen. Protect from light.

(continued)

(Daunorubicin citrate liposome injection continued)

DRUG ADMINISTRATION

IV bolus over 60 minutes, repeated every 2 weeks.

Do not use an inline filter.

Drug is an irritant, not a vesicant.

Dose should be reduced in patients with renal or hepatic dysfunction.

Hold dose if absolute granulocyte count is < 750 cells/mm^3.

SPECIAL CONSIDERATIONS

Drug is embryotoxic, so female patients should use contraceptive measures as appropriate.

Back pain, flushing, and chest tightness may occur during the first 5 minutes of drug administration and resolve with cessation of the infusion. Most patients do not experience recurrence when the infusion is restarted at a slower rate.

Drug indicated in the treatment of Kaposi's sarcoma. Activity reported to be equivalent to treatment with ABV (doxorubicin, vincristine, bleomycin) but with less alopecia, cardiotoxicity, and neurotoxicity.

Daunorubicin citrate liposome injection

Nursing Diagnosis	Defining Characteristics
I. *Potential for infection and bleeding related to bone marrow depression*	I. A. Myelosuppression can be severe and affects the granulocytes primarily B. Incidence of neutropenia—36% C. Neutropenia with < 500 cells/mm³ occurs in 15% of pts
II. *Alteration in comfort related to back pain, flushing, chest tightness*	II. A. Occurs in 13.8% of pts and is mild to moderate B. The syndrome resolves with cessation of the infusion, and does not usually recur when the infusion is resumed at a slower infusion rate
III. *Potential for alteration in skin integrity related to alopecia, changes in skin*	III. A. Mild alopecia occurs in 6% of pts and moderate alopecia in 2% of pts

Expected Outcomes	Nursing Interventions
I. A. Pt will be without s/s of infection or bleeding	I. A. Monitor Hct, WBC with differential, and platelets prior to drug administration. Discuss any abnormalities with physician (drug should not be given if ANC is < 750 cells/mm³)
B. Signs of infection and/or bleeding will be identified and reported early	B. Drug dose to be reduced with renal impairment: if creatinine is greater than 3 mg/dl, reduce dose by 50%
	C. Drug dose to be reduced with hepatic dysfunction: 50% reduction if serum bilirubin is greater than 3mg/dl, 25% reduction if serum bilirubin is 1.2–3.0 mg/dl
	D. Assess for s/s infection and bleeding, and instruct pt in self-assessment and to report s/s immediately
	E. Teach pt self-care measures to minimize risk of infection and bleeding, including avoidance of OTC aspirin-containing medications
II. A. Pt will report comfort throughout infusion	II. A. Infuse drug at prescribed rate (over 60 mins); assess for, and teach pt to report, back pain, flushing, and chest tightness
	B. Stop infusion if any of the above occur; resume infusion at a slower rate once symptoms subside
III. A. Pt's skin will remain intact	III. A. Teach pt about small chance of hair loss and measures to cope with it, should it occur
	B. Teach pt that hair loss is uncommon

Daunorubicin citrate liposome injection *(continued)*

Nursing Diagnosis	Defining Characteristics
IV. *Potential for alteration in nutrition, less than body requirements, related to nausea and vomiting, anorexia, diarrhea*	IV. A. Mild nausea occurs in 35% of pts, moderate nausea in 16% of pts, and severe nausea in 3% of pts B. Vomiting is less common C. Anorexia may occur (21%) or increased appetite may occur in < 5% of pts D. Diarrhea occurs in 38% of pts. Other GI problems, occurring < 5% of the time, are dysphagia, gastritis, hemorrhoids, hepatomegaly, dry mouth, and tooth caries
V. *Potential for alteration in cardiac output related to cardiac changes*	V. A. Daunorubicin may cause cardiotoxicity and CHF, but studies with liposomal daunorubicin show rare clinical cardiotoxicity at cumulative doses > 600 mg/m^2

Expected Outcomes	**Nursing Interventions**

IV. A. Pt will be without nausea or vomiting
      B. Nausea and vomiting, should they occur, will be minimal
      C. Pt's weight will remain within 5% of baseline
	IV. A. Premedicate with antiemetics. Encourage small, frequent feedings of cool, bland foods
	      B. If pt has anorexia, teach patient or caregiver to make foods ahead of time, use spices, and encourage weekly weights
	      C. Encourage pt to report diarrhea, and to use self-management strategies (medications as ordered, diet modifications)
	      D. Instruct patient to report other GI symptoms

V. A. Pt will maintain baseline cardiac function	V. A. Assess cardiac status prior to chemotherapy administration (esp. in patients with preexisting cardiac disease or prior anthracycline treatment). Tests may include s/s CHF, quality, regularity and rate of heartbeat, results of prior tests of left ventricular ejection fraction (LVEF) or echocardiogram, if performed
	      B. Instruct pt to report dyspnea, palpitations, swelling in extremities
	      C. Maintain accurate records of total dose, and expect GBPS to be repeated periodically during treatment
	      D. Testing of cardiac function should be performed at cumulative doses of 320 mg/m^2, 480 mg/m^2, and every 240 mg/m^2 thereafter

Docetaxel
(Taxotere)

Class: Taxoid, mitotic spindle poison

MECHANISM OF ACTION

Enhances microtubule assembly and inhibits tubulin depolymerization, thus arresting cell division in metaphase. Cell cycle-specific
for M-phase.

METABOLISM

Drug is extensively protein-bound (94–97%). Triphasic elimination
when infused over 1–2 hours. Metabolism appears to involve P-
450 3A (CYP3A4) isoenzyme system (in vitro testing). Fecal elimination is main route, accounting for excretion of 75% of the drug
within 7 days; 80% of the fecal excretion occurred during the first
48 hours. Mild to moderate liver impairment (SGOT+/or SGPT >
1.5 times normal and alk phos > 2.5 times normal) results in delayed metabolism of drug by 27%, resulting in a 38% increase in
systemic exposure (AUC).

DOSAGE/RANGE

Breast cancer: 60–100 mg/m^2 IV as a 1-hour infusion every 3 weeks

Non-small-cell-lung-cancer: 75 mg/m^2 as a 1-hour infusion every 3
weeks

Premedication regime with corticosteroids: e.g., dexamethasone 8 mg
bid × 3 days, starting 1 day prior to docetaxel to reduce risk of
fluid retention and hypersensitivity reactions.

DRUG PREPARATION

Vials available as 80 mg/2 ml (40 mg/ml) and 20 mg/0.5 ml, also (40 mg/ml) single-dose vials in blister packs with diluent.

Unopened vials require refrigeration and protection from bright light. Allow to stand at room temperature for 5 minutes prior to reconstitution.

Reconstitute 20-mg and 80-mg vials with accompanying diluent (13% ethanol in water for injection).

Use only glass or polypropylene or polyolefin plastic (bag) IV containers.

Withdraw ordered dose, and further dilute in 250 ml of 5% dextrose or 0.9% sodium chloride for a final concentration of 0.3–0.9 mg/ml. If the dose exceeds 240 mg of docetaxel, use a larger volume of diluent to achieve a final concentration of < 0.9 mg/ml.

Inspect for any particulate matter or discoloration, and, if found, discard.

Reconstituted vials (premix solution) stable for 8 hours at either room temperature or refrigeration.

DRUG ADMINISTRATION

Assess patient's ANC, and treat only if ANC > 1500/mm^3; assess liver function studies and if abnormality, discuss with physician. See Special Considerations.

Use only glass or polypropylene bottles, or polypropylene or polyolefin plastic bags for drug infusion, and administer infusion ONLY through polyethylene-lined administration sets.

Patient should receive corticosteroid premedication (e.g., dexamethasone 8 mg bid) for 3 days beginning 1 day before drug administration to reduce the incidence and severity of fluid retention and hypersensitivity reactions.

Administer drug infusion over 1 hour.

(continued)

(Docetaxel continued)

SPECIAL CONSIDERATIONS

Indicated for the treatment of (1) locally advanced or metastatic breast cancer after failure of prior chemotherapy, and (2) locally advanced or metastatic non-small-cell lung cancer (NSCLC) after failure of prior platinum-based chemotherapy.

Contraindicated in patients with history of severe hypersensitivity reactions to docetaxel or to other drugs formulated with polysorbate 80; drug should not be used in patients with neutrophil counts of < 1500 cells/mm^3. Drug should not be used in pregnant or breast-feeding women; women of child-bearing age should use effective birth control measures.

Radiosensitizing effect

Theoretically, CYP3A4 inhibitors such as ketoconazole, erythromycin, troleandomycin, cyclosporine, terfenadine, and nifedipine can inhibit docetaxel metabolism and result in elevated serum levels of docetaxel; use together with caution or not at all.

Theoretically, CYP3A4 inducers, such as anti-convulsants and St. John's Wort, may increase metabolism and decrease serum levels of docetaxel.

Docetaxel generally should not be administered to patients with bilirubin > upper limit of normal (ULN) or to patients with SGOT and/or SGPT > 1.5 × ULN concomitant with alkaline phosphatase > 2.5 × ULN. Patients treated with elevated bilirubin or abnormal transaminases plus alkaline phosphatase have an increased risk of grade 4 neutropenia, febrile neutropenia, severe stomatitis, infections, severe thrombocytopenia, severe skin toxicity, and toxic death. Serum bilirubin, SGOT or SGPT, and alkaline phosphatase should be obtained and reviewed by the treating physician before each cycle of docetaxel treatment.

Dose modifications during treatment: (1) Patients with breast cancer dosed initially at 100 mg/m^2 who experience either febrile neutropenia, ANC < 500/mm^3 for > 1 week, or severe or cumulative cutaneous reactions, should have dose reduced to 75 mg/m^2. If reactions continue at the reduced dose, further reduce to 55 mg/m^2 or discontinue drug. Patients dosed initially at 60 mg/m^2 who do not experience febrile neutropenia. ANC < 500/mm^3 for > 1 week, severe cutaneous reactions, or severe peripheral neuropathy during drug therapy may tolerate higher drug doses and may be dose-escalated. Patients who develop > grade 3 peripheral neuropathy should have drug discontinued; (2) Patients with NSCLC dosed initially at 75 mg/m^2 who experience either febrile neutropenia, ANC < 500 mg/m^2 for > 1 week, severe or cumulative cutaneous reactions, or other nonhematologic toxicity grades 3 or 4 should have treatment withheld until toxicity resolves, and then have dose reduced to 55 mg/m^2; patients who develop > grade 3 peripheral neuropathy should discontinue docetaxel chemotherapy.

Patients should receive 3-day dexamethasone premedication.

Administration of docetaxel in Europe is not subject to United States Federal Drug Administration recommendations—non-PVC containers and tubing are not required.

Incomplete cross-resistance between paclitaxel and docetaxel in many tumor types.

Studies ongoing to determine effectiveness of docetaxel 30–45 mg/m^2 weekly in metastatic breast cancer, as drug given in this fashion may act as antiangiogenesis agent, and also provides "dose-dense" therapy, which provides less opportunity for malignant cells to develop resistant clones. Weekly dose schedules being studied are 3 weeks of treatment, one week off, or 6 weeks of treatment, and 2 weeks off, with drug being administered as a 30-minute infusion. Most common side effects when drug is given this way are asthenia, anemia, fluid retention, nail toxicity, and hyperlacrimation. Corticosteroid premedication is often dexamethasone 4 or 8 mg po q 12 hours × 3 doses beginning day before treatment.

Docetaxel

Nursing Diagnosis	Defining Characteristics
I. *Infection and bleeding related to bone marrow depression*	I. A. Neutropenia is dose-limiting toxicity B. Thrombocytopenia is less frequent
II. *Potential for injury related to hypersensitivity reactions*	II. A. Hypersensitivity reactions usually occur with initial treatment, if at all

Expected Outcomes	Nursing Interventions

I.   A. Pt will be without s/s of infection and bleeding
    B. Early s/s of infection or bleeding will be identified
	I. A. Monitor WBC, platelet count prior to drug administration and periodically after treatment
	    B. Monitor pt for s/s of infection or bleeding and teach pt self-assessment and how to seek medical advice/care
	    C. Drug dose should be reduced or held for low blood values

II. A. Early s/s of hyper-sensitivity reactions will be identified	II. A. Review standing orders for management of hypersensitivity reactions and identify location of anaphylaxis kit containing epinephrine 1:1000, hydrocortisone sodium succinate (SoluCortef), diphenhydramine HCl (Benadryl), Aminophylline, and other medications
	    B. Prior to drug administration, obtain baseline vital signs and record mental status assessment
	      1. Premedicate with diphenhydramine and dexamethasone as ordered
	      2. Assess pt for at least 30 mins after the drug is given for s/s of a reaction
	      3. Teach pt to report any hypersensitivity reactions or unusual symptoms
	    C. Observe for the following s/s during infusion, usually occurring within first 15 mins of start of infusion:
	      1. *Subjective*
	        a. Generalized itching
	        b. Nausea
	        c. Chest tightness
	        d. Crampy abdominal pain
	        e. Difficulty speaking
	        f. Anxiety
	        g. Agitation
	        h. Sense of impending doom

Docetaxel *Continued*

Nursing Diagnosis	Defining Characteristics
II. *Potential for injury related to hypersensitivity reactions*	
III. *Potential impairment of skin integrity related to* A. Rash	III. A. Maculopapular, violaceous rash may occur

Expected Outcomes	Nursing Interventions

	i. Uneasiness
	    j. Desire to urinate or defecate
	      k. Dizziness
	      l. Chills
	  2. *Objective*
	    a. Flushed appearance (angioedema of face, lips, neck, eyelids, hands)
	    b. Localized or generalized urticaria
	    c. Respiratory distress $\pm$ wheezing
	    d. Hypotension
	    e. Cyanosis
	D. If reaction occurs, stop infusion and notify MD
	E. Place pt in supine position to promote perfusion of visceral organs
	F. Monitor vital signs until stable
	G. Provide emotional support to patient and family
	H. Maintain pt airway and have equipment for CPR close by
	I. Document incident and pt response to treatment
	J. Discuss with MD desensitization and increased premedication for future treatments

III. A. Pt will verbally report skin rash and describe self-care measures	III. A. 1. Assess skin for any cutaneous changes, such as rash, and any associated symptoms, such as pruritus; discuss with MD
	      2. Instruct patient in self-care measures
	        a. Avoiding abrasive skin products, clothing
	        b. Avoiding tight-fitting clothing
	        c. Use of skin emollients appropriate for skin alteration
	        d. Measures to avoid scratching involved areas

Docetaxel *Continued*

Nursing Diagnosis	Defining Characteristics
B. Alopecia	B. Alopecia may occur
IV. *Potential alterations in fluid and electrolyte balance*	IV. A. Peripheral edema and pleural effusions may occur

Expected Outcomes	Nursing Interventions
B. Pt will verbalize feelings re hair loss and strategies to cope with change in body image	B. 1. Discuss potential impact of hair loss prior to drug administration, coping strategies, and plan to minimize body image distortion (e.g., wig, scarf, cap) 2. Assess pt for s/s of hair loss 3. Assess pts response and use of coping strategies
IV. A. Edema or effusions will be identified early	IV. A. Assess baseline skin turgor, especially extremities B. Assess respiratory status, including breath sounds C. Teach pt to report any alterations in breathing patterns D. Discuss abnormal findings with MD

Doxorubicin hydrochloride
(Adriamycin, Rubex)

Class: Anthracycline antibiotic isolated from streptomycin products, in particular from the rhodomycin products

MECHANISM OF ACTION

Antitumor antibiotic—no clearly defined mechanism. Binds directly to DNA base pairs (intercalates) and inhibits DNA and DNA-dependent RNA synthesis, as well as protein synthesis. Cell cycle-specific for S phase.

METABOLISM

Excretion of drug predominates in the liver; renal clearance is minor. Drug excreted through urine and may discolor urine 1–48 hours after administration.

DOSAGE/RANGE

30–75 mg/m^2 IV every 3–4 weeks
20–45 mg/m^2 IV for 3 consecutive days
For bladder instillation: 3–60 mg/m^2
For intraperitoneal instillation: 40 mg in 2 liters dialysate (no heparin)
Continuous infusion: varies with individual protocol

DRUG PREPARATION

Drug will form a precipitate if mixed with heparin or 5-fluorouracil. Dilute with sodium chloride (preservative-free) to produce 2 mg/ml concentration.

DRUG ADMINISTRATION

Give IV push through the sidearm of a freely flowing IV or as a bolus
over 1–2 hours or as a continuous infusion over 24 hours. Must
be given via a central line if given via bolus or continuous infusion, as drug is a potent vesicant.

SPECIAL CONSIDERATIONS

Drug is a potent vesicant. Give through running IV to avoid extravasation and tissue necrosis.

Give through central line if drug is to be given by continuous infusion.

Causes discoloration of urine (from pink to red) for up to 48 hours.

Skin changes: may cause "recall phenomenon"—recalls reaction to
previously irradiated tissue.

Cardiac toxicity: dose limit at 550 mg/m^2. Patients may exhibit irreversible CHF. May see acute toxicity in hours or days after administration. This is unrelated to cumulative dose and may manifest
symptoms of pump or conduction function. Rarely, transient EKG
abnormalities, CHF, pericardial effusions (whole syndrome referred to as myocarditis-pericarditis syndrome) may occur, which
may lead to demise of patient.

Vein discoloration.

Increased pigmentation in black patients.

When given with barbiturates, there is increased plasma clearance of
doxorubicin.

When given with cyclophosphamide, there is risk of hemorrhage and
cardiotoxicity.

When given with mitomycin, there is increased risk of cardiotoxicity.

There is decreased oral bioavailability of digoxin when given together.

When given with mercaptopurine, there is increased risk of hepatotoxicity.

Abnormalities in liver function require dose modification.

Doxorubicin hydrochloride

Nursing Diagnosis	Defining Characteristics
I. *Potential for infection and bleeding related to bone marrow depression*	I. A. Nadir 10–14 days, with recovery 15–21 days B. Myelosuppression may be severe; overall incidence 60–80%, less common with weekly dosing
II. *Potential for alteration in nutrition, less than body requirements* A. Nausea and vomiting	II. A. 1. Moderate to severe; 50% incidence as single agent, with increased incidence in combination with Cytoxan 2. Onset 1–3 hrs after drug administration, lasting up to 24 hrs
B. Anorexia	B. Occurs frequently
C. Stomatitis	C. 10% incidence esophagitis
III. *Potential for alteration in cardiac output*	III. A. Acute: pericarditis-myocarditis syndrome with nonspecific EKG changes (flat T waves, ST, PVCs) during infusion or immediately after (non-life threatening) B. Cumulative dose cardiomyopathy; risk if dose > 550 mg/m^2 or > 450 mg/m^2 when receiving chest XRT or Cytoxan

Expected Outcomes	Nursing Interventions

I.   A. Pt will be without s/s of infection or bleeding
    B. Early s/s of infection or bleeding will be identified
	I. A. 1. Monitor CBC, platelet count prior to drug administration, as well as s/s of infection and bleeding
	      2. Instruct pt in self-assessment of s/s of infection and bleeding
	      3. Dose reduction may be necessary; discuss with MD
	      4. Transfuse with red cells and platelets per MD order
	      5. Administer growth factors as ordered

II.   A. 1. Pt will be without nausea and vomiting
      2. Nausea and vomiting, if they occur, will be minimal
 	
    B. Pt will maintain baseline weight ± 5%
 	
    C. Oral mucous membrane will remain intact and without infection
	II. A. 1. Premedicate with antiemetics and continue prophylactically × 24 hrs to prevent nausea and vomiting, at least first treatment
	      2. Encourage small, frequent feedings of cool, bland foods and liquids
	    B. 1. Encourage small, frequent feedings of favorite foods, especially high-calorie, high-protein foods
	      2. Encourage use of spices
	      3. Weekly weights
	    C. 1. Teach pt oral assessment
	      2. Encourage pt to report early signs of stomatitis

III. A. Early s/s of cardio-myopathy will be identified	III. A. If pt is receiving cyclophosphamide in addition to doxorubicin, assess for s/s of cardiomyopathy
	    B. Cardiac evaluation on a regular basis
	    C. Discuss gated blood pool scans with MD, baseline and periodically
	    D. Assess pts baseline cardiac function prior to beginning chemotherapy
	    E. Assess quality and regularity of heartbeat

Doxorubicin hydrochloride *Continued*

Nursing Diagnosis	Defining Characteristics
III. *Potential for alteration in cardiac output*	
IV. *Potential for sexual dysfunction*	IV. A. Drug is teratogenic and mutagenic

V. *Alteration in skin integrity*
  A. Alopecia
	V. A. Complete hair loss with 60–75 mg/m^2 dosing
	    1. Occurs 2–5 weeks after therapy begins
	    2. Regrowth usually begins a few month after drug is stopped

B. Changes in nails and skin, radiation recall reaction, flare reaction	B. 1. Nail beds and dermal creases (especially in black patients) become hyperpigmented
	    2. Reactivation of the erythema and skin damage of prior sites of skin irradiation
	    3. Erythematous streaking along vein during drug administration, often with urticaria and pruritus; this condition is self-limiting, usually within 30 mins with or without use of antihistamines

C. Extravasation	C. Avoid extravasation, as tissue necrosis may occur

Expected Outcomes	Nursing Interventions
	F. Instruct pt to report dyspnea, shortness of breath
IV. A. Pt and significant other will understand need for contraception	IV. A. As appropriate, explore with pt and significant other reproductive and sexuality pattern and impact chemotherapy will have
B. Pt and significant other will identify strategies to cope with sexual dysfunction	B. Discuss strategies to preserve sexuality and reproductive health
V. A. Pt will verbalize feelings re hair loss and identify strategies to cope with change in body image	V. A. 1. Assess pt for s/s of hair loss 2. Discuss with pt impact of hair loss and strategies to minimize distress (e.g., wig, scarf, cap)
B. Pt will verbalize feelings re changes in nail or skin color or texture and identify strategies to cope with change in body image	B. 1. Assess pt for changes in skin and nails 2. Discuss with pt impact of changes and strategies to minimize distress (e.g., wearing nail polish or long sleeves)
C. 1. Extravasation, if it occurs, will be detected early, with early intervention 2. Skin and underlying tissue damage will be minimized	C. 1. Use careful technique during venipuncture 2. Administer vesicant through freely flowing IV, constantly monitoring IV site and patient response 3. Nurse should be *thoroughly* familiar with institutional policy and procedure for administration of a vesicant agent 4. If vesicant drug is administered as a continuous infusion, drug must be given through a patent central line

Doxorubicin hydrochloride   *Continued*

Nursing Diagnosis	Defining Characteristics
C. Extravasation	

Expected Outcomes	**Nursing Interventions**

	5. If extravasation is suspected:
	  a. Stop drug being administered
	  b. Aspirate any residual drug and blood from IV tubing, IV catheter/needle, and IV site if possible
	  c. *If antidote exists,* instill antidote into area of apparent infiltration as per MD order and institutional policy and procedure
	  d. Apply cold or topical medication as per MD order and institutional policy and procedure
	6. Assess site regularly for pain, progression of erythema, induration, and evidence of necrosis
	7. When in doubt about whether drug is infiltrating, *treat as an infiltration*
	8. Teach pt to assess site and notify MD if condition worsens
	9. Arrange next clinic visit for assessment of site depending on drug, amount infiltrated, extent of potential injury, and patient variables
	10. Document in pt record as per institutional policy and procedure

Etoposide
(VP-16, Vepesid)

Class: Plant alkaloid, a derivative of the mandrake plant (mayapple plant)

MECHANISM OF ACTION

Inhibits DNA synthesis in S and G_2 so that cells do not enter mitosis. Causes single-strand breaks in DNA. Cell cycle–specific for S and G_2 phases.

METABOLISM

VP-16 is rapidly excreted in the urine and, to a lesser extent, the bile. About 30% of drug is excreted unchanged. Binds to serum albumin (94%), then becomes extensively tissue bound.

DOSAGE/RANGE

50–100 mg/m^2 IV qd × 5 (testicular cancer) q 3–4 weeks
75–200 mg/m^2 IV qd × 3 (small-cell lung cancer) q 3–4 weeks
Oral dose is twice intravenous dose.

DRUG PREPARATION

Available in 5 cc (100 mg) vials
Oral capsules available in 50-mg and 100-mg capsules

DRUG ADMINISTRATION

IV infusion: over 30–60 minutes to minimize risk of hypotension and bronchospasm (wheezing). In some instances, a test dose may be infused slowly (0.5 ml in 50 NS) and the remaining drug infused if no untoward reaction after 5 minutes.

Stability: drug must be diluted with either 5% dextrose injection, USP, or 0.9% sodium chloride solution and is stable 96 hours in glass and 48 hours in plastic containers at room temperature (77°F, 25°C) under normal fluorescent light at a concentration of 0.2 mg/ml.

Inspect for clarity of solution prior to administration.

Oral administration: may give as a single dose if $\leq$ 400 mg; otherwise divide dose.

SPECIAL CONSIDERATIONS

Reduce drug dose by 50% if bilirubin $>$ 1.5 mg/dl, by 75% if bilirubin $>$ 3.0 mg/dl.

Synergistic drug effect in combination with cisplatin.

Radiation recall may occur when combined therapies are used.

Etoposide

Nursing Diagnosis	Defining Characteristics
I. *Potential for injury during drug administration related to*	I.
A. Allergic reaction	A. Bronchospasm as evidenced by wheezing may occur; may experience fever, chills
B. Hypotension	B. Hypotension may occur during rapid infusion
C. Anaphylaxis	C. Anaphylaxis may occur but is rare

Expected Outcomes	**Nursing Interventions**

I. A. 1. Bronchospasm will be prevented
     2. Bronchospasm, if it occurs, will be identified early and terminated
 	
   B. Hypotension will be prevented
	I. A. 1. Infuse drug slowly over at least 30–60 mins
	     2. Discontinue drug and notify MD if bronchospasm occurs; have antihistamines ready (e.g., diphenhydramine)
	
	   B. 1. Monitor BP prior to drug administration and periodically during infusion, at least during first drug administration
	     2. Infuse drug over *at least* 30–60 mins; slow rate of infusion if BP drops

C. Anaphylaxis, if it occurs, will be managed successfully	C. 1. Monitor pt closely during infusion
	    2. Review standing orders for management of pt in anaphylaxis and identify location of anaphylaxis kit containing epinephrine 1:1000, hydrocortisone sodium succinate (SoluCortel), diphenhydramine HCL (Benadryl), Aminophylline, and others
	    3. Prior to drug administration, obtain baseline vital signs and record mental status
	    4. Observe for following s/s during infusion, usually occurring within first 15 mins of start of infusion
	       a. *Subjective*
	          (1) generalized itching
	          (2) nausea
	          (3) chest tightness
	          (4) crampy abdominal pain
	          (5) difficulty speaking
	          (6) anxiety
	          (7) agitation

Etoposide *Continued*

Nursing Diagnosis	Defining Characteristics
C. Anaphylaxis	
II. *Potential for infection and bleeding related to bone marrow depression*	II. A. Nadir 7–14 days B. Dose-limiting toxicity C. Granulocytopenia can be severe D. Neutropenia, thrombocytopenia, anemia can all occur E. Recovery 20–22 days

Expected Outcomes	**Nursing Interventions**
	(8) sense of impending doom
	(9) uneasiness
	(10) desire to urinate or defecate
	(11) dizziness
	(12) chills
	b. *Objective*
	(1) flushed appearance (angioedema of face, neck, eyelids, hands, feet)
	(2) localized or generalized urticaria
	(3) respiratory distress ± wheezing
	(4) hypotension
	(5) cyanosis
	5. Stop infusion if reaction occurs and notify MD
	6. Place pt in supine position to promote perfusion of visceral organs
	7. Monitor vital signs until stable
	8. Provide emotional reassurance to pt and family
	9. Maintain patent airway and have CPR equipment ready if needed
	10. Document incident
	11. Discuss with MD desensitization versus drug discontinuance for further dosing
II. A. Pt will be without s/s of infection or bleeding B. Early s/s of infection or bleeding will be identified	II. A. Monitor CBC, platelet count prior to drug administration and at time of expected nadir B. Assess for s/s of infection and bleeding C. Instruct pt in self-assessment of s/s of infection and bleeding

Etoposide *Continued*

Nursing Diagnosis	Defining Characteristics
II. *Potential for infection and bleeding related to bone marrow depression*	
III. *Altered nutrition, less than body requirements related to* A. Nausea and vomiting	III. A. 1. Usually mild, occurring soon after infusion 2. Intensity and frequency increase with oral dosing and may be severe
B. Anorexia	B. Usually mild but may be severe with oral dosing
IV. *Body image disturbance related to alopecia*	IV. A. Incidence 20–90% depending on dose; regrowth may occur between drug cycles
V. *Potential for sexual dysfunction*	V. A. Drug is teratogenic and embryocidal in rats B. Drug is mutagenic

Expected Outcomes	Nursing Interventions
	D. Dose reduction may be necessary with compromised bone marrow function, low nadir counts, or hepatic dysfunction

III. A. 1. Pt will be without nausea and vomiting
         2. If nausea and vomiting occur, they will be minimal
	III. A. 1. Premedicate with antiemetics and continue prophylactically for at least 4–6 hrs after drug administration, at least first treatment
	            2. Encourage small, frequent feedings of cool, bland foods and liquids

B. Pt will maintain weight within ± 5% baseline	B. 1. Encourage small, frequent feedings of favorite foods, especially high-calorie, high-protein foods
	         2. Encourage use of spices
	         3. Weekly weights in ambulatory setting

IV. A. Pt will verbalize feelings re hair loss and identify strategies to cope with change in body image	IV. A. Discuss with pt anticipated impact of hair loss; suggest wig as appropriate prior to actual hair loss B. Explore with pt response to hair loss and strategies used to minimize distress (e.g., wig, scarf, cap)
V. A. Pt and significant other will understand need for contraception	V. A. As appropriate, explore with pt and significant other issues of reproductive and sexual patterns and expected impact chemotherapy will have
B. Pt and significant other will identify strategies to cope with sexual dysfunction	B. Discuss strategies to preserve sexuality and reproductive health (e.g., sperm banking, contraception)

Etoposide *Continued*

Nursing Diagnosis	Defining Characteristics
VI. *Altered skin integrity related to* A. Radiation recall	VI. A. Radiation sensitizer: may reactivate skin reactions from prior radiation therapy
B. Irritation	B. Perivascular irritation may occur if drug extravasates
VII. *Alteration in cardiac output*	VII. A. Rare B. Myocardial infarction has been reported after prior mediastinal XRT and in pts receiving VP-16-containing combination chemotherapy C. Arrhythmias have been reported but are rare
VIII. *Sensory/perceptual alterations related to neurological toxicities*	VIII. A. Peripheral neuropathies may occur but are rare and mild

Expected Outcomes	Nursing Interventions
VI. A. Skin surface will remain intact or heal following injury	VI. A. 1. Assess skin in area of prior XRT when combined therapies are given 2. If radiation recall results in skin breakdown, drug may need to be withheld until skin healing occurs 3. Wound management based on type of skin reaction
B. Skin irritation will be minimal	B. 1. Use careful venipuncture techniques and administer drug over 30–60 mins, diluted as directed by manufacturer
VII. A. Early cardiac dysfunction will be identified	VII. A. Monitor pt closely during treatment, especially with coexisting cardiac dysfunction B. Notify MD of any abnormalities C. Document any irregular cardiac rhythm on EKG
VIII. A. Peripheral neuropathies will be identified early B. Pt will verbalize feelings re discomfort and dysfunction related to neuropathies and will identify alternate coping strategies	VIII. A. Assess motor and sensory function prior to therapy B. Encourage pt to verbalize feelings re discomfort and sensory loss if these occur C. Assist pt to discuss alternative coping strategies

Fludarabine phosphate
(Fludara, FLAMP)

Class: Antimetabolite

MECHANISM OF ACTION

Interferes with DNA synthesis by inhibiting ribonucleotide reductase.

METABOLISM

Rapidly converted to the active metabolite 2-fluoroara-A (2-FLAA). About 23% of the dose is excreted as 2-FLAA over 5 days.

DOSAGE/RANGE

20–30 mg/m^2 IV over 30 minutes daily for 5 days. Cycle resumes every 28 days except with bone marrow or other toxicity

or

20 mg/m^2 loading dose (bolus), then 30 mg/m^2 continuous infusion for 48 hours

DRUG PREPARATION

50-mg vial. Reconstitute with 2 ml sterile water. Discard unused solutions after 8 hours, as drug contains no preservative.

DRUG ADMINISTRATION

Administer as an IV bolus or continuous infusion.

SPECIAL CONSIDERATIONS

Use drug with caution in patients with advanced age, renal insufficiency, bone marrow impairment, or neurological deficiency.

Severe risk of pulmonary toxicity when fludarabine is given with pentostatin.

May cause tumor lysis syndrome (TLS). Hydrate and use allopurinol to prevent TLS.

Do not use in patients with known hypersensitivity to fludarabine.

Fludarabine phosphate

Nursing Diagnosis	Defining Characteristics
I. *Infection and bleeding related to bone marrow depression*	I. A. Anemia, thrombocytopenia, neutropenia occur, with nadir at 13 days B. Bone marrow fibrosis and hemolytic anemia may occur C. Myelosuppression is the dose-limiting toxicity
II. *Alteration in nutrition, less than body requirements related to* A. Nausea and vomiting	II. A. Nausea, vomiting, diarrhea occur in 30% of pts
B. Stomatitis	B. Stomatitis and GI bleeding
C. Anorexia	C. Anorexia

Expected Outcomes	**Nursing Interventions**
I. A. Pt will be without s/s of infection or bleeding	I. A. Monitor CBC, platelet count prior to drug administration B. Monitor for s/s of infection and bleeding C. Instruct pt in self-assessment of s/s of infection and bleeding D. Transfuse with RBCs, platelets per MD order
II. A. 1. Pt will be without nausea and vomiting 2. Pt will maintain weight within 5% of baseline	II. A. 1. Premedicate with antiemetics and continue prophylactically × 24 hrs to prevent nausea and vomiting, at least for first treatment 2. Encourage small, frequent feedings of cool, bland foods and liquids 3. I&O, daily weights if inpatient (assess for s/s of fluid and electrolyte imbalance)
B. Mucous membranes of GI tract will remain intact	B. 1. Assess oral cavity every day; teach pt to do own oral assessment and oral hygiene regimen 2. Encourage pt to report early stomatitis 3. Pain relief measures if indicated
C. Pt will maintain baseline weight ± 5%	C. 1. Encourage small, frequent feedings of favorite foods, especially high-calorie, high-protein foods 2. Encourage use of spices 3. Weekly weights 4. Dietary consult as needed

Fludarabine phosphate *Continued*

Nursing Diagnosis	Defining Characteristics
III. *Potential impaired gas exchange related to pulmonary toxicity*	III. A. Pulmonary toxicity can include dyspnea, cough, fever, hypoxia, interstitial pulmonary infiltrates, effusions B. Onset is 3–28 days after third to fifth cycle
IV. *Potential alteration in cardiac output*	IV. A. Pericardial effusion and edema sometimes occur
V. *Potential for sensory/ perceptual alterations related to neurological toxicity*	V. A. CNS neurotoxicity can include weakness, headache, confusion, agitation, visual disturbances, hearing loss, coma B. Peripheral paresthesias

Expected Outcomes	Nursing Interventions
III. A. Early s/s of pulmonary toxicity will be identified	III. A. Discuss with MD the need for pulmonary function tests and CXR prior to beginning therapy B. Assess lung sounds prior to drug administration C. Instruct pt to report cough, dyspnea, shortness of breath
IV. A. Pt will maintain vital signs within normal limits	IV. A. Monitor vital signs, especially BP; listen for pulsus paradoxus, an indication of possible cardiac tamponade B. Cardiac evaluation as needed
V. A. S/s of neurotoxicity will be identified early	V. A. Monitor for s/s of neurotoxicity before and during each treatment B. Teach pt about possible neurotoxicity and s/s

5-Fluorouracil
(Fluorouracil, Adrucil, 5-FU, Efudex [topical])

Class: Pyrimidine antimetabolite

MECHANISM OF ACTION

Acts as a "false" pyrimidine, inhibiting the formation of an enzyme (thymidine synthetase) necessary for the synthesis of DNA. Also incorporates into RNA, causing abnormal synthesis. Methotrexate given prior to 5-fluorouracil results in synergism and enhanced efficacy.

METABOLISM

Metabolized by the liver. Most is excreted as respiratory CO_2; remainder is excreted by the kidneys. Plasma half-life is 20 minutes.

DOSAGE/RANGE

12–15 mg/kg IV once a week

or

12 mg/kg IV every day × 5 days every 4 weeks

or

500 mg/m² every week or every week × 5

Hepatic infusion: 22 mg/kg in 100 ml D_5W infused into hepatic artery over 8 hours for 5–21 consecutive days

Head and neck: 1000 mg/m² day as continuous infusion for 4–5 days

DRUG PREPARATION

No dilution required. Can be added to NS or D_5W.

Store at room temperature; protect from light. Solution should be clear. If crystals do not disappear after holding vial under hot water, discard vial.

DRUG ADMINISTRATION

Given IV push or bolus (slow drip) or as continuous infusion.

Given topically as cream.

SPECIAL CONSIDERATIONS

Patients who have had adrenalectomy may need higher doses of prednisone while receiving 5-FU, or dose of 5-FU may be reduced in postadrenalectomy patients.

Reduce dose in patients with compromised hepatic, renal, or bone marrow function and malnutrition.

Inspect solution for precipitate prior to continuous infusion.

When given with cimetidine, there are increased pharmacologic effects of fluorouracil.

When given with thiazide diuretics, there is increased risk of myelosuppression.

5-Fluorouracil

Nursing Diagnosis	Defining Characteristics
I. *Altered nutrition, less than body requirements related to* A. Nausea and vomiting	I. A. Occur occasionally, may last 2–3 days, usually preventable with antiemetics

B. Stomatitis	B. 1. Onset 5–8 days
	        2. May herald severe bone marrow depression
	        3. Indication to interrupt therapy

C. Diarrhea	C. 1. Indication to interrupt treatment 2. May occur with esophagopharyngitis—sore throat with dysphagia

II. *Infection and bleeding related to bone marrow depression*	II. A. Common
	     B. Neutropenia, thrombocytopenia are most significant
	     C. Nadir 7–14 days after first dose

Expected Outcomes	**Nursing Interventions**

I. A. 1. Pt will be without nausea or vomiting
      2. Nausea and vomiting, if they occur, will be minimal
	I. A. 1. Premedicate with antiemetics and continue prophylactically × 24 hrs to prevent nausea and vomiting, at least with the first treatment
	      2. Encourage small, frequent feedings of cool, bland foods and liquids
	      3. Assess for s/s of fluid and electrolyte imbalance: monitor I&O and daily weights if inpatient

B. Oral mucous membranes will remain intact and free of infection	B. 1. Assess mouth prior to each dose; stomatitis is sometimes preceded by a beefy, painful tongue or small, shallow ulcers on the inner lip
	      2. Report stomatitis to MD; may need to interrupt therapy
	      3. Teach pt oral assessment and mouth care
	      4. Use pain relief measures

C. 1. Pt will have minimal diarrhea
      2. Early s/s of esophagopharyngitis will be identified and treated
	C. 1. Encourage pt to report onset of diarrhea
	      2. Administer or teach pt to self-administer antidiarrheal medication
	      3. Guaiac all stools
	      4. Encourage adequate hydration
	      5. Assess pt for sore throat, dysphagia
	      6. Treat with topical anesthetics

II. A. Pt will be without s/s of infection or bleeding	II. A. Monitor CBC, platelet count prior to drug administration, as well as as s/s of infection and bleeding
B. Early s/s of infection or bleeding will be identified	B. Instruct pt in self-assessment of s/s of infection and bleeding

5-Fluorouracil *Continued*

Nursing Diagnosis	Defining Characteristics

III. *Alteration in skin integrity related to*
     A. Alopecia
	III. A. 1. More common with 5-day course of treatment; uncommon with 1-day course
	           2. Diffuse thinning, loss of eyelashes and eyebrows

B. Changes in nails and skin	B. 1. Nail loss and brittle cracking of nails may occur
	           2. Photosensitivity/photophobia may occur
	           3. Maculopapular rash sometimes occurs on the extremities and trunk (rarely serious); hyperpigmentation on the palms of hands, face
	           4. Chemical phlebitis may occur during continuous infusions, related to high pH of drug

IV. *Sensory perceptual alterations*	IV. A. Occasional cerebellar ataxia (reversible when drug is discontinued)
	      B. Somnolence
	      C. Ocular changes: conjunctivitis, increased lacrimation, photophobia, oculomotor dysfunction, blurred vision
	      D. Occasional euphoria

Expected Outcomes	Nursing Interventions
III. A. Pt will verbalize feelings re hair loss and identify strategies to cope with change in body image	III. A. 1. Assess pt for s/s of hair loss 2. Discuss with pt impact of hair loss and strategies to minimize distress (e.g., wig, scarf, cap); begin before therapy is initiated
B. Pt will verbalize feelings re changes in nails and skin and identify strategies to cope with change in body image	B. 1. Assess pt for changes in nails and skin 2. Discuss with pt impact of changes and strategies to minimize distress (e.g., wearing nail polish or long sleeves) 3. Instruct pt in importance of staying out of sun or wearing sunscreen if sun exposure is unavoidable 4. Assess skin for rash or other changes; report changes to MD (pt may need antihistamines or steroids) 5. Consider implanted venous access device and discuss with pt and physician
IV. A. Early neurological changes will be identified B. Pt will identify strategies for coping with neurological changes	IV. A. Assess cerebellar function prior to each treatment B. Teach pt safety precautions as needed C. Assess pt for ocular changes; report changes

Flutamide
(Eulexin)

Class: Antiandrogen

MECHANISM OF ACTION

Exerts its effect by inhibiting androgen uptake or by inhibiting nuclear
binding of androgen in target tissues or both.

METABOLISM

Rapidly and completely absorbed. Excreted mainly via urine. Biolog-
ically active metabolite reaches maximum plasma levels in approximately 2 hours. Plasma half-life is 6 hours. Largely plasma
bound.

DOSAGE/RANGE

250 mg every 8 hours

DRUG PREPARATION

Available in 125-mg tablets

DRUG ADMINISTRATION

Oral

SPECIAL CONSIDERATIONS

None

Flutamide

Nursing Diagnosis	Defining Characteristics
I. *Alteration in comfort*	I. A. Hot flashes occur commonly
II. *Sexual dysfunction*	II. A. Causes decreased libido and impotence in about a third of pts B. Gynecomastia occurs in about 10% of pts
III. *Altered nutrition, less than body requirements related to* A. Diarrhea B. Nausea and vomiting	III. A. Occurs in about 10% of pts B. Occurs in about 10% of pts

Expected Outcomes	Nursing Interventions

I. A. Pt will be without hot flashes
    B. Discomfort will be identified and treated early
	I. A. Inform pt that hot flashes may occur
	    B. Encourage pt to report symptoms early

II. A. Pt and significant other will verbalize understanding of changes in sexuality and body image that may occur	II. A. As appropriate, explore with pt and significant other issues of reproductive and sexuality patterns and the impact chemotherapy may have on them B. Discuss strategies to preserve sexuality and reproductive health

III. A. 1. Pt will have minimal diarrhea
 	
    B. 1. Pt will be without nausea and vomiting
      2. Nausea and vomiting, should they occur, will be minimal
	III. A. 1. Encourage pt to report onset of diarrhea
	      2. Administer or teach pt to self-administer antidiarrheals
	      3. Guaiac stools
	    B. 1. Inform pt of possibility of nausea and vomiting. Obtain prescription for antiemetic if necessary
	      2. Encourage small, frequent feedings of cool, bland foods

Gemcitabine
(difluorodeoxycitidine, dFdC)

Class: Antimetabolite

MECHANISM OF ACTION

Structurally similar to Ara-C. Inhibits DNA synthesis by inhibiting DNA polymerase activity. Cell cycle-specific for S phase, causing cells to accumulate at the G-S boundary.

METABOLISM

Metabolized by enzymes in tumor cells. Cleared renally.

DOSAGE/RANGE

Current recommendation for phase II trials is 800–1000 mg/m^2 weekly for 3 weeks, with the cycle repeating every 4 weeks

or

Given at dose of 3600 mg/m^2 every 2 weeks

DRUG PREPARATION

Reconstitute with 2 ml NS (for 20-mg vial) or 10 ml NS (for 100-mg vial).

Further dilute in NS. Drug dose of 2500 mg/m^2 or more must be diluted in at least 1000 ml NS and infused over 4 hours or longer.

DRUG ADMINISTRATION

Most commonly infused over 30 minutes weekly. Doses over 2500 mg/m^2 must be infused over at least 4 hours.

SPECIAL CONSIDERATIONS

Peripheral (ankle) edema sometimes occurs.

Gemcitabine

Nursing Diagnosis	Defining Characteristics
I. *Potential for bleeding related to bone marrow depression*	I. A. Thrombocytopenia is dose-limiting toxicity B. Relatively little leukopenia seen, rare anemia C. Myelosuppression resolves rapidly when drug is discontinued
II. *Potential alteration in comfort*	II. A. Flu-like symptoms with transient febrile episodes occur in 50% of pts with first dose only B. 1. Skin rash (occasionally) within 2–3 days of starting drug 2. Erythematous, pruritic, maculopapular rash of the neck and extremities
III. *Potential alteration in nutrition, less than body requirements*	III. A. Nausea and vomiting mild; respond to conventional antiemetics

Expected Outcomes	Nursing Interventions

I.   A. Pt will remain free of s/s of bleeding
    B. Hematocrit will be maintained at greater than 25, platelets at greater than 10,000
	I. A. Monitor CBC, platelet count prior to drug administration, as well as s/s of infection and bleeding
	    B. Instruct pt in self-assessment of s/s of infection and bleeding
	    C. Transfuse with red cells, platelets per MD order

II. A. Pt will report absence of flu-like symptoms
    B. Skin rash will be identified and treated early
	II. A. 1. Encourage pt to report flu-like symptoms
	       2. Treat fevers with acetaminophen
	    B. 1. Treat rash with topical corticosteroids
	       2. Discuss with MD possible dose reductions to avoid rash with subsequent administration

III. A. Nausea and vomiting will be prevented	III. A. Treat nausea and vomiting with conventional antiemetics
	    B. Premedicate with antiemetics and continue prophylactically × 24 hrs to prevent nausea and vomiting, at least for first treatment
	    C. Encourage small, frequent feedings of cool, bland foods and liquids
	    D. I&O, daily weights if inpt (assess for s/s of fluid and electrolyte imbalance)

Hydroxyurea
(Hydrea)

Class: Miscellaneous/antimetabolite

MECHANISM OF ACTION

Antimetabolite that prevents conversion of ribonucleotides to de-oxyribonucleotides by inhibiting the converting enzyme ribonu-cleoside diphosphate reductase. DNA synthesis is thus inhibited. Cell cycle phase-specific—S phase. May also sensitize cells to the effects of radiation therapy, although the process is not clearly understood.

METABOLISM

Rapidly absorbed from gastrointestinal tract.

Peak plasma level reached in 2 hours, with plasma half-life of 3–4 hours. About half the drug is metabolized in the liver, half ex-creted in urine as urea and unchanged drug. Some of the drug is eliminated as respiratory CO_2. Crosses blood-brain barrier.

DOSAGE/RANGE

20–30 mg/kg/day orally as a continuous dose

50–75 mg/kg/day IV

DRUG PREPARATION

Available in 500-mg capsules

DRUG ADMINISTRATION

Oral

SPECIAL CONSIDERATIONS

Hydroxyurea has a side effect of dramatically lowering WBC in a relatively short period of time (24–48 hours). In leukemia patients endangered by the potential complication of leukostasis, this is the desired effect.

May need to pretreat with allopurinol to protect patient from tumor lysis syndrome.

Dermatologic radiation recall phenomena may occur.

In combination with radiation therapy, mucosal reactions in the radiation field may be severe.

Hydroxyurea

Nursing Diagnosis		Defining Characteristics	
I.	*Infection and bleeding related to bone marrow depression*	I.	A. Leukopenia more common than thrombocytopenia B. WBC may start dropping in 24–48 hrs; nadir seen in 10 days, with recovery within 10–30 days C. Severity of leukopenia is dose related
II.	*Altered nutrition, less than body requirements related to* A. Anorexia	II.	A. Mild to moderate
	B. Stomatitis		B. Uncommon
	C. Diarrhea		C. Uncommon
	D. Hepatic dysfunction		D. Hepatitis is rare but may occur; there are also disturbances in liver function studies
III.	*Alteration in skin integrity related to* A. Alopecia	III.	A. Uncommon, though may be slight to diffuse thinning

Expected Outcomes	**Nursing Interventions**
I. A. Pt will be without s/s of infection or bleeding B. Early s/s of infection or bleeding will be identified	I. A. Monitor CBC, platelet count prior to drug administration as well as s/s of infection or bleeding B. Instruct pt in self-assessment of infection or bleeding C. Drug dosage may be titrated for higher or lower than normal blood values
II. A. Pt will maintain baseline weight ± 5% B. Oral mucous membranes will remain intact and without infection C. Pt will have minimal diarrhea D. Hepatic dysfunction will be identified early	II. A. 1. Encourage small, frequent feedings of favorite foods, especially high-calorie, high-protein foods 2. Encourage use of spices 3. Weekly weights B. 1. Teach pt oral assessment and mouth care 2. Encourage pt to report early stomatitis 3. Teach pt oral hygiene C. 1. Encourage pt to report onset of diarrhea 2. Administer or teach pt to self-administer antidiarrheal medications D. 1. Monitor SGOT, SGPT, LDH, alkaline phosphatase, and bilirubin periodically during treatment 2. Notify MD of any elevations
III. A. Pt will verbalize feelings re hair loss and identify strategies to cope with change in body image	III. A. 1. Assess pt for s/s of hair loss 2. Discuss with pt impact of hair loss and strategies to minimize distress (i.e., wig, scarf, cap); begin before therapy is initiated

Hydroxyurea *Continued*

Nursing Diagnosis	Defining Characteristics
B. Dermatitis	B. 1. Dermatitis is uncommon, usually mild and reversible 2. Symptoms may include facial erythema, rash pruritus 3. Rarely, postirradiation therapy erythema (recall) may occur
IV. *Alteration in renal function related to chemotherapy (rare)*	IV. A. Reversible renal tubular dysfunction evidenced by elevated BUN, creatinine, and uric acid levels
V. *Potential for sexual/ reproductive dysfunction*	V. A. Gonadal function and fertility are affected (may be permanent or transient) B. Reported to be excreted in breast milk reproductive dysfunction
VI. *Sensory/perceptual alterations*	VI. A. S/s may include disorientation, drowsiness headache, vertigo B. Symptoms usually do not last more than 24 hrs

Expected Outcomes	**Nursing Interventions**
B. 1. Skin will remain intact 2. Early skin impairment will be identified	B. 1. Assess skin integrity 2. If dermatitis severe, discuss drug discontinuance with MD 3. Topical medications as appropriate 4. Radiation recall occurs when hydroxyurea is administered during or after radiation therapy and may occur weeks or months after therapy
IV. A. Pt will be without renal dysfunction	IV. A. Monitor BUN and creatinine prior to drug dose, as half of drug is excreted unchanged in urine B. Provide or instruct pt in hydration of *at least* 2–3 liters of fluid/day during and for at least 48 hrs after therapy C. Monitor I&O D. Weekly weights
V. A. Pt. and significant other will understand need for contraception B. Pt and significant other will identify strategies to cope with sexual and reproductive dysfunction	V. A. As appropriate, explore with pt and significant other issues of reproductive and sexuality pattern and impact chemotherapy will have B. Discuss strategies to preserve sexuality and reproductive health (e.g., contraception, sperm banking)
VI. A. Mental status changes and other disturbances will be identified early	VI. A. Obtain baseline mental status—neurological function B. Assess status changes during chemotherapy C. Encourage pt to report any changes

Idarubicin
(Idamycin, 4-Demethoxydaunorubicin)

Class: Antitumor antibiotic

MECHANISM OF ACTION

Cell cycle phase-specific for S phase. Analogue of daunorubicin. Has a
marked inhibitory effect on RNA synthesis.

METABOLISM

Excreted primarily in the bile and to a lesser extent the urine, with approximately 25% of the IV dose accounted for over 5 days. The
half-life of this agent and its metabolite is 18–50 hours.

DOSAGE/RANGE

12 mg/m^2 daily × 3 days by slow IVB (over 10–15 minutes) in combination with Ara-C 100 mg/m^2 IV continuous infusion for 7 days
or
25 mg/m^2 IVB followed by Ara-C 200 mg/m^2 continuous infusion
daily for 5 days

DRUG PREPARATION

Available as a red powder. The drug is reconstituted with normal
saline injection.

DRUG ADMINISTRATION

Drug is a vesicant. Administer IV push over 10–15 minutes into the sidearm of a freely running IV.

SPECIAL CONSIDERATIONS

Vesicant.

Discolored urine (pink to red) may occur up to 48 hours after administration.

Cardiomyopathy is less common and less severe than with doxorubicin and daunorubicin.

Drug is light sensitive.

Incompatible with heparin (precipitate occurs).

Drug dosage should be reduced in patients with hepatic or renal dysfunction.

Idarubicin

Nursing Diagnosis		Defining Characteristics
I.	*Infection and bleeding related to bone marrow depression*	I. A. Hematologic toxicity is dose limiting B. Leukopenia nadir 10–20 days, with recovery in 1–2 weeks C. Thrombocytopenia usually follows leukopenia and is mild D. BM toxicity is not cumulative
II.	*Altered nutrition, less than body requirements related to* A. Nausea and vomiting	II. A. Usually mild to moderate, though nausea and vomiting are seen to some degree in most pts
	B. Anorexia	B. Commonly occurs
	C. Stomatitis	C. Mild
	D. Diarrhea	D. Infrequent and mild
	E. Hepatic dysfunction	E. 1. Hepatitis is rare but may occur 2. There are also disturbances in liver function studies

Expected Outcomes	**Nursing Interventions**
I. A. Pt will be without s/s of infection or bleeding B. Early s/s of infection or bleeding will be identified C. Administer growth factors (esp. GCSF) as ordered	I. A. Monitor CBC, platelet count prior to drug administration as well as s/s of infection or bleeding B. Instruct pt in self-assessment of s/s of infection or bleeding C. Dose modifications often necessary (35–50%) if bone marrow function is compromised

II. A. 1. Pt will be without nausea and vomiting
    2. Nausea and vomiting, if they occur, will be minimal
 	
B. Pt will maintain baseline weight ± 5%
 	
C. Oral mucous membranes will remain intact and without infection
 	
D. Pt will have minimal diarrhea
 	
E. Hepatic dysfunction will be identified early
	II. A. 1. Premedicate with antiemetics and continue prophylactically × 24 hrs to prevent nausea and vomiting, at least first treatment
	    2. Encourage small, frequent feedings of cool, bland foods and liquids
	B. 1. Encourage small, frequent feedings of favorite foods, especially high-calorie, high-protein foods
	    2. Encourage use of spices
	    3. Weekly weights
	C. 1. Teach pt oral assessment and mouth care
	    2. Encourage pt to report early stomatitis
	    3. Teach pt oral hygiene
	D. 1. Encourage pt to report onset of diarrhea
	    2. Administer or teach pt to self-administer antidiarrheal medications
	E. 1. Monitor SGOT, SGPT, LDH, alkaline phosphatase, and bilirubin periodically during treatment
	    2. Notify MD of any elevations

Idarubicin *Continued*

Nursing Diagnosis	Defining Characteristics
III. *Alteration in skin integrity related to* A. Alopecia	III. A. 1. Occurs in about 30% of pts after oral drug and can be partial after IV drug 2. Begins after 3 + weeks, and hair may grow back while on therapy 3. May be slight to diffuse thinning
B. Skin changes: darkening of nail beds, skin ulcer/ necrosis, sensitivity to sunlight, skin itching at irradiated areas	B. Skin changes seen as hyperpigmentation of nail beds, sensitivity to sunlight, radiation recall, and potential necrosis with extravasation

Expected Outcomes	**Nursing Interventions**
III. A. Pt will verbalize feelings re hair loss and identify strategies to cope with change in body image	III. A. 1. Assess pt for s/s of hair loss 2. Discuss with pt impact of hair loss and strategies to minimize distress (e.g., wigs, scarf, cap); begin before therapy is initiated

B. 1. Skin will remain intact
2. Early skin impairment will be identified
	B. 1. Assess skin for integrity
	2. If severe, discuss drug discontinuance with MD
	3. Assess pt for changes in skin, nails
	4. Discuss with pt impact of changes and strategies to minimize distress (e.g., wearing nail polish, long sleeves)
	5. Administer according to policies for vesicant drugs
	  a. Use careful technique during venipuncture
	  b. Administer vesicant through freely flowing IV, constantly monitoring IV site and pt response
	  c. Nurse should be *thoroughly* familiar with institutional policy and procedure for administration of a vesicant agent
	  d. If vesicant drug is administered as a continuous infusion, drug must be given through a patent central line
	  e. If extravasation is suspected:
	    (1) stop drug being administered
	    (2) aspirate any residual drug and blood from IV tubing, IV catheter/needle, and IV site if possible

Idarubicin   *Continued*

Nursing Diagnosis	Defining Characteristics
B. Skin changes: darkening of nail beds, skin ulcer/ necrosis, sensitivity to sunlight, skin itching at irradiated areas	B. Skin changes seen as hyperpigmentation of nail beds, sensitivity to sunlight, radiation recall, and potential necrosis with extravasation
IV. *Alteration in cardiac output related to cumulative doses*	IV. A. Cardiac toxicity is similar characteristically but less severe than that seen with daunorubicin and doxorubicin B. CHF due to cardiomyopathy seen after large cumulative doses

Expected Outcomes	**Nursing Interventions**
	(3) *if antidote exists,* instill antidote into area of apparent infiltration as per MD order and institutional policy and procedure
	(4) apply cold or topical medications as per MD order and institutional policy and procedure
	f. Assess site regularly for pain, progression of erythema, induration, and evidence of necrosis
	g. When in doubt about whether drug is infiltrating, *treat as an infiltration*
	h. Teach pt to assess site and notify MD if condition worsens
	i. Arrange next clinic visit for assessment of site depending on drug, amount infiltrated, extent of potential injury, and pt variables
	j. Document in pt record as per institutional policy and procedure
IV. A. Early s/s of cardiomyopathy will be identified	IV. A. Assess pt for s/s of cardiomyopathy
	B. Obtain baseline cardiac functions (EKG changes uncommon)
	C. Discuss gated blood pool scan or echocardiogram with MD
	D. Assess quality and regularity of heartbeat
	E. Instruct pt to report dyspnea, shortness of breath
	F. Teach pt the potential of irreversible CHF with cumulative doses

Ifosfamide
(IFEX)

Class: Alkylating agent

MECHANISM OF ACTION

Analogue of cyclophosphamide and is cell cycle phase-nonspecific. Destroys DNA throughout the cell cycle by binding to protein and DNA, cross-linking with DNA and causing chain scission as well as inhibition of DNA synthesis. Ifosfamide has been shown to be effective in tumors previously resistant to cyclophosphamide. Activated by microsomes in the liver.

METABOLISM

Only about 50% of the drug is metabolized, with much of the drug excreted in the urine almost completely unchanged. Half-life is 13.8 hours for high dose versus 3–10 hours for lower doses.

DOSAGE/RANGE

IV bolus 50 mg/kg/day
or
700–2000 mg/m^2/day × 5 days
or
2400 mg/m^2/day × 3 days
Continuous infusion: 1200 mg/m^2/day × 5 days
Single dose: 5000 mg/m^2 q 3–4 weeks
Dose reduce by 25–50% if serum creatinine is 2.1–3.0 mg/dl

DRUG PREPARATION

Available as a powder and should be reconstituted with sterile water for injection.

Solution is chemically stable for 7 days, but discard after 8 hours due to lack of bacteriostatic preservative of the solution.

May be diluted further in either D_5W or normal saline.

DRUG ADMINISTRATION

IV bolus: administer over 30 minutes.

Continuous infusion: administer IV for 5 days. Mesna should be administered with ifosfamide: it is begun simultaneously with the drug and repeated at 4 and 8 hours after the ifosfamide. (See drug sheet on mesna.) Mesna, ascorbic acid, and Mucomyst have been utilized to protect the bladder. Prehydration and posthydration (150–2000 cc/day) or continuous bladder irrigations are recommended to prevent hemorrhagic cystitis.

SPECIAL CONSIDERATIONS

Metabolic toxicity is increased by simultaneous administration of barbiturates.

Activity and toxicity of the drug may be altered by allopurinol, chloroquine, phenothiazines, potassium iodide, chloramphenicol, imipramine, vitamin A, corticosteroids, and succinylcholine.

Therapy requires the concomitant administration of a uroprotector such as mesna and prehydration and posthydration; may also require catheterization and constant bladder irrigation, and/or ascorbic acid.

Ifosfamide

Nursing Diagnosis	Defining Characteristics
I. *Altered urinary elimination related to*	
A. Hemorrhagic cystitis	I. A. 1. Symptoms of bladder irritation 2. Hemorrhagic cystitis with hematuria, dysuria, urinary frequency 3. Preventable with uroprotection and hydration
B. Renal toxicity	B. 1. Symptoms of renal toxicity 2. ↑ BUN, ↑ serum creatinine, ↓ urine creatinine clearance (usually reversible) 3. Acute tubular necrosis, pyelonephritis, glomerular dysfunction 4. Metabolic acidosis
II. *Altered nutrition, less than body requirements* A. Nausea and vomiting	II. A. 1. Nausea and vomiting occur in 58% of pts 2. Dose and schedule dependent; ↑ severity with higher dose and rapid injection 3. Occurs within a few hours of drug administration and may last 3 days

Expected Outcomes	**Nursing Interventions**
I. A. 1. Pt will be without hemorrhagic cystitis 2. Hemorrhagic cystitis, if it occurs, will be detected early	I. A. 1. Assess presence of RBC in urine prior to successive doses, especially if symptoms are present, as well as BUN and creatinine 2. Administer drug with concomitant uroprotector (e.g., mesna) 3. Encourage *prehydration:* po intake of 2–3 1/day prior to chemotherapy; *posthydration:* increase po fluids to 2–3 1/day for 2 days after chemotherapy 4. If possible, administer drug in morning to minimize drug accumulation in bladder during sleep 5. Instruct pt to empty bladder every 2–3 hours, before bedtime, and during night when awake 6. Monitor urinary output and total body balance
B. Renal dysfunction will be identified early	B. 1. Assess urinary elimination pattern prior to each drug dose 2. If rigorous regimen is adhered to, minimal renal toxicity will result 3. Monitor BUN and creatinine 4. IV hydration as ordered 5. Drug dose should be reduced if serum creatinine 2.1–3.0 mg/dl. Hold drug if > 3.0
II. A. 1. Pt will be without nausea and vomiting 2. Nausea and vomiting, if they occur, will be minimal	II. A. 1. Premedicate with antiemetics and continue prophylactically to *prevent* nausea and vomiting for 24 hrs, at least first treatment 2. Encourage small, frequent feedings of cool, bland foods and liquids

Ifosfamide *Continued*

Nursing Diagnosis	Defining Characteristics
B. Hepatotoxicity	B. 1. Elevations of serum transaminase and alkaline phosphatase may occur 2. Usually transient and resolves spontaneously 3. No apparent sequelae
III. *Infection and bleeding related to bone marrow depression*	III. A. Leukopenia is mild to moderate B. Thrombocytopenia and anemia are rare C. Bone marrow depression more severe when ifosfamide is combined with other chemotherapy agents D. Pts at risk for BMD: pts with impaired renal function and bone marrow reserve (bone marrow metastases, prior XRT)
IV. *Alteration in skin integrity related to* A. Alopecia	IV. A. Incidence 83%, with 50% experiencing severe hair loss in 2–4 weeks
B. Sterile phlebitis at injection site; irritation with extravasation	B. Drug is not activated until it reaches hepatic microsomes, so drug doesn't cause tissue damage (is not a vesicant); incidence < 2%
C. Skin changes	C. Skin hyperpigmentation, dermatitis, nail ridging may occur

Expected Outcomes	Nursing Interventions
B. Early hepatotoxicity will be identified	B. Monitor LFTs during treatment; report elevation to MD
III. A. Pt will be without s/s of infection or bleeding B. Early s/s of infection or bleeding will be identified	III. A. Monitor CBC, platelet count prior to drug administration, as well as s/s of infection or bleeding B. Instruct pt in self-assessment of s/s of infection or bleeding C. Dose reduction may be necessary when given in combination with other agents causing BMD
IV. A. Pt will verbalize feelings re hair loss and identify strategies to cope with change in body image B. 1. Skin injury will be prevented 2. Early injury will be identified C. 1. Early skin impairment will be identified 2. Pt will verbalize feelings re changes in nail or skin color or texture and identify strategies to cope with change in body image	IV. A. 1. Discuss with pt anticipated impact of hair loss; suggest wig, as appropriate, prior to actual hair loss 2. Explore with pt response to hair loss and alternative strategies to minimize distress B. Carefully monitor injection site during drug administration and infusion for s/s of phlebitis, irritation, vein patency C. 1. Assess skin integrity 2. Assess impact of skin changes on body image 3. Discuss strategies to minimize distress

Ifosfamide *Continued*

Nursing Diagnosis	Defining Characteristics
V. *Sensory/perceptual alterations: confusion, activity intolerance, fatigue*	V. A. Intact drug passes easily into CNS; however, *active* metabolites do not B. Lethargy and confusion may be seen with high doses, lasting 1–8 hours; usually spontaneously reversible C. CNS side effects occur in about 12% of pts treated, including somnolence, confusion, depressive psychosis, hallucinations D. Less frequent: dizziness, disorientation, cranial nerve dysfunction, seizures E. Incidence of CNS side effects may be higher in pts with compromised renal function, as well as in pts receiving high dose
VI. *Potential for sexual dysfunction*	VI. A. Drug is carcinogenic, mutagenic, and teratogenic B. Drug is excreted in breast milk

Expected Outcomes	Nursing Interventions

V. A. Neurologic alterations will be identified early
 	
    B. Pt and family will manage distress safely
	V. A. Identify pts at risk ($\downarrow$ renal function) and observe closely
	    B. Assess neurological and mental status prior to and during drug administration and on follow-up
	    C. Instruct pt to report any alterations in behavior, sensation, perception
	    D. If side effects develop, create a plan of care with pt and family to manage distress and promote safety

VI. A. Pt and significant other will understand need for contraception
 	
    B. Pt and significant other will identify strategies to cope with sexual dysfunction
	VI. A. As appropriate, explore with pt and significant other issues of reproductive and sexual pattern and impact chemotherapy will have
	    B. Discuss strategies to preserve sexuality and reproductive health (e.g., sperm banking, contraception)

Irinotecan
(Camptosar, Camptothecin-11, CPT-11)

Class: Topoisomerase inhibitor

MECHANISM OF ACTION

Induces protein-linked DNA single-strand breaks and blocks DNA and RNA synthesis in dividing cells, preventing cells from entering mitosis. Prevents DNA repair.

METABOLISM

Metabolized to active metabolite SN-38 in the liver; 11–20% of drug excreted in urine, and 5–39% in the bile, over a 48-hour period. Mean terminal half-life is 6 hours, while that of SN-38 is 10 hours. Drug is moderately protein-bound (30–68%) while SN-38 is highly protein-bound (95%).

DOSAGE/RANGE

Starting dose is 125 mg/m^2 IV over 90 minutes weekly × 4, followed by 2-week rest period. Repeat 6-week cycle.

If well-tolerated, dose can be increased to 150 mg/m^2.

350 mg/m^2 IV day/repeated q 3 weeks has same efficacy (300 mg/m^2 if age ≥ 70, prior pelvic/ abdominal XRT, or performance status of 2).

Drug combined with 5FU and leucovorin is more active than 5FU/ leucovorin alone.

DRUG PREPARATION

Store at room temperature protected from light.
Dilute and mix drug in 5% glucose solution.

DRUG ADMINISTRATION

Administer IV bolus over 90 minutes.

SPECIAL CONSIDERATIONS

Drug is indicated for treatment of metastatic colon or rectal cancer recurring or progressing after 5FU treatment.

Dose-limiting toxicities are diarrhea and severe myelosuppression.

Drug is synergistic with cisplatin; give irinotecan *after* cisplatin to maximize cell kill.

Drug is teratogenic and contraindicated in pregnant women.

Drug is an irritant; if infiltration occurs, manufacturer recommends flushing IV site with sterile water, and then applying ice.

All patients should receive self-care instruction on management of diarrhea, self-administration of loperamide for delayed diarrhea, and accurate assessment of the patient's ability to purchase and take loperamide if diarrhea develops.

Dose reduce for neutropenia and diarrhea.

Response to therapy usually evaluable after 2 cycles.

Drug active in other solid tumors, including non-small cell lung cancer.

Irinotecan

Nursing Diagnosis	Defining Characteristics
I. *Potential for infection, fatigue related to bone marrow depression*	I. A. Leukopenia has been noted in 50–60% of pts on the single-dose schedule B. Anemia reported in 15% of pts
II. *Potential alteration in bowel elimination pattern related to diarrhea*	II. A. Diarrhea common and may occur during or immediately after treatment (cholinergic response). Often associated with diaphoresis, abdominal cramping; preventable by IV atropine 0.25 mg IV B. Delayed diarrhea occurs day 8–13, may be severe and requires compliance to antidiarrheal medicines
III. *Alteration in nutrition related to nausea and vomiting*	III. A. Nausea and vomiting mod–severe B. Occurs in 35–60% of pts C. Preventable using serotonin antagonist antiemetic therapy

Expected Outcomes	**Nursing Interventions**
I. A. Pt is without s/s of infection	I. A. 1. Monitor CBC, platelet count prior to drug administration, as well as s/s of infection and bleeding 2. Instruct pt in self-assessment of s/s of infection and bleeding 3. Transfuse with platelets per MD order
B. Pt reports ability to participate in normal ADLs	B. 1. Check hematocrit; transfuse with RBCs per MD order 2. Instruct pt in energy conservation measures
II. A. Diarrhea will be prevented	II. A. Assess normal bowel elimination status, ability to manage self-care and ability to purchase loperamide
B. Diarrhea, if it occurs, will be managed effectively	B. Ensure patient understands required self-administration of loperamide if diarrhea develops C. Teach pt to administer Immodium, 2 tabs after first episode of diarrhea then 1 tab q 2 hrs until no diarrhea × 12 hours (at bedtime, take 2 tabs) (recommended by Camptosar manufacturer) D. Teach pt to modify diet to eliminate fiber, fruits/vegetables that cause diarrhea, to eat small, frequent meals, try BRAT diet, increase po fluids.
III. A. Pt will be without nausea and vomiting	III. A. Premedicate with antiemetics and continue prophylactically × 24 hrs to prevent nausea and vomiting, at least for first treatment
B. Pt will maintain weight within 5% of baseline	B. Encourage small, frequent feedings of cool, bland foods and liquids C. Monitor I&O, total body balance, electrolyte balance D. Teach pt self-administration of antiemetics at home, and to report if they are ineffective

Irinotecan   *Continued*

Nursing Diagnosis	Defining Characteristics
IV. *Alteration in skin integrity*	IV. A. Alopecia occurs in 30–40% of pts
V. *Potential impaired gas exchange related to pulmonary toxicity*	V. A. Diffuse interstitial infiltrates have occurred in 8% of pts with fever and dyspnea B. Interstitial pneumonitis rare

Expected Outcomes	Nursing Interventions
IV. A. Pt verbalizes feelings about hair loss and identifies strategies to cope with change in body image	IV. A. Assess pt for hair loss B. Discuss with pt impact of hair loss and strategies to minimize distress (e.g., scarf, cap, wig)
V. A. Pt will maintain baseline pulmonary function	V. A. Discuss with MD the need for pulmonary function tests and CXR prior to beginning therapy B. Assess lung sounds prior to drug administration C. Instruct pt to report cough, dyspnea, shortness of breath D. Administer glucocorticoids as directed

L-asparaginase
(ELSPAR)

Class: Miscellaneous/enzyme

MECHANISM OF ACTION

Hydrolysis of serum asparagine occurs, which deprives leukemia cells of the required amino acid. Normal cells are spared because they generally have the ability to synthesize their own asparagine.

Cell cycle-specific for G_1 postmitotic phase.

Some leukemic cells are unable to synthesize asparagine. These cells must obtain asparagine from an exogenous source—the patient's serum. Administration of the enzyme L-asparaginase causes hydrolysis of asparagine to aspartate, resulting in rapid depletion of the asparagine concentration in the patient's serum.

METABOLISM

Metabolism of L-asparaginase is independent of renal and hepatic function. The drug is not recovered in the urine and does not appear to cross the blood-brain barrier.

DOSAGE/RANGE

IM or IV, varies with protocol

DRUG PREPARATION

IV injection: Reconstitute with sterile water for injection or sodium chloride injection (without preservative) and use within 8 hours of reconstitution.

IV infusion: Dilute with sodium chloride injection or 5% dextrose injection and use within 8 hours, only if clear; if gelatinous particles develop, filter through a 5-micron filter.

The lyophilized powder must be stored under refrigeration. The reconstituted solution must also be stored under refrigeration if it is not used immediately. The solution must be discarded within 8 hours after preparation.

DRUG ADMINISTRATION

Use in a hospital setting. Make preparations to treat anaphylaxis at each administration of the drug.

SPECIAL CONSIDERATIONS

Potential reduction in antineoplastic effect of methotrexate when given in combination.

Anaphylaxis is associated with the administration of this drug.

Intravenous administration of L-asparaginase concurrently with or immediately before prednisone and vincristine administration may be associated with increased toxicity.

L-asparaginase

Nursing Diagnosis	Defining Characteristics

I. *Potential for injury related to hypersensitivity or anaphylactic reaction*	I. A. Occurs in 20–35% of pts
	B. Increased incidence after several doses administered but may occur with first dose
	C. Occurs less often with IM route of administration
	D. May be life-threatening reaction but usually mild
	   1. Urticardial eruptions
	   2. Fever (100°–101°F, 37.5°–38°C) seen in half of pts
	   3. Chills
	   4. Facial redness
	   5. Hypotension
	   6. Shortness of breath
	   7. Hives
	   8. Diaphoresis

Expected Outcomes	Nursing Interventions

I. A. Early s/s of hypersensitivity or anaphylactic reactions will be identified	I. A. Teach pt the potential of a hypersensitivity or anaphylaxis reaction and to immediately report any unusual symptoms
	B. Obtain baseline vital signs and note pt's mental status
	C. Skin testing, prior to administering full dose, is recommended by manufacturer
	D. Assess pt for at least 30 mins after the drug is given for s/s of a reaction
	E. 1. Administer therapy according to MD orders
	    2. Review standing orders for management of pt in anaphylaxis and identify location of anaphylaxis kit containing epinephrine 1:1000, hydrocortisone sodium succinate (Solucortef), diphenhydramine HCl (Benadryl), Aminophylline, and others
	    3. Observe for following s/s during infusion, usually occurring within first 15 mins of start of infusion
	      a. *Subjective*
	        (1) generalized itching
	        (2) nausea
	        (3) chest tightness
	        (4) crampy abdominal pain
	        (5) difficulty speaking
	        (6) anxiety
	        (7) agitation
	        (8) sense of impending doom
	        (9) uneasiness
	       (10) desire to urinate/defecate
	       (11) dizziness
	       (12) chills

L-asparaginase   *Continued*

Nursing Diagnosis	Defining Characteristics
I. *Potential for injury related to hypersensitivity or anaphylactic reaction*	
II. *Altered nutrition, less than body requirements related to* A. Nausea and vomiting	II. A. 50–60% of pts experience mild to severe nausea and vomiting starting within 4–6 hrs after treatment

Expected Outcomes	Nursing Interventions

	b. *Objective*
	       (1) flushed appearance (angioedema of face, neck, eyelids, hands, feet)
	       (2) localized or generalized urticaria
	       (3) respiratory distress ± wheezing
	       (4) hypotension
	       (5) cyanosis
	  4. If reaction occurs, stop infusion and notify MD
	  5. Place pt in supine position to promote perfusion of visceral organs
	  6. Monitor vital signs until stable
	  7. Provide emotional reassurance to pt and family
	  8. Maintain patent airway and have CPR equipment ready if needed
	  9. Document incident
	  10. Discuss with MD desensitization versus drug discontinuance for further dosing
	F. *Escherichia coli* preparation of L-asparaginase and *Erwinia carotovora* preparation are non-cross-resistant, so if an anaphylaxis reaction occurs with one, the other preparation may be used

Expected Outcomes	Nursing Interventions

I. A. 1. Pt will be without nausea and vomiting
    2. Nausea and vomiting, if they occur, will be minimal
	II. A. 1. Premedicate with antiemetics and continue prophylactically × 24 hrs to prevent nausea and vomiting
	    2. Encourage small, frequent feedings of cool, bland foods and liquids

L-asparaginase *Continued*

Nursing Diagnosis	Defining Characteristics
B. Anorexia	B. Commonly occurs
C. Hyperglycemia	C. 1. Transient reaction caused by effects on the pancreas 2. ↓ insulin synthesis 3. Pancreatitis in 5% of pts
III. *Hepatic dysfunction or thromboembolic potential*	III. A. Two-thirds of pts have elevated LFTs starting within first 2 weeks of treatment (i.e., SGOT, bilirubin, alkaline phosphatase) B. Hepatically derived clotting factors may be depressed, resulting in excessive bleeding or blood clotting; relatively uncommon
IV. *Mental status alteration*	IV. A. 25% of pts experience some changes in mental status—commonly lethargy, drowsiness, and somnolence; rarely coma B. Predominantly seen in adults C. Malaise occurs in most pts and generally gets worse with subsequent doses D. Drug does not cross blood-brain barrier

Expected Outcomes	Nursing Interventions
B. Pt will maintain baseline weight ± 5%	B. 1. Encourage small, frequent feedings of favorite foods, especially high-calorie, high-protein foods 2. Encourage use of spices 3. Weekly weights
C. 1. Pt will be without s/s of hyperglycemia or pancreatitis 2. Early s/s of hyperglycemia or pancreatitis will be identified	C. 1. Teach pt the potential of hyperglycemia and pancreatitis and to report any unusual symptoms (i.e., increased thirst, urination, and appetite) 2. Monitor serum glucose, amylase, and lipase levels periodically during treatment 3. Report any laboratory elevations to MD 4. Treat hyperglycemia issues with diet or insulin as ordered by MD 5. Treat pancreatitis per MD orders
III. A. Hepatic dysfunction will be identified early	III. A. Monitor SGOT, bilirubin, alkaline phosphatase, albumin, and clotting factors—PT, PTT, fibrinogen B. Teach pt the potential of excessive bleeding or blood clotting and to report any unusual symptoms C. Assess pt for s/s of bleeding or thrombosis
IV. A. Pt will be without changes in mental status (e.g., depression)	IV. A. Teach pt of the potential of CNS toxicity and to report any unusual symptoms B. Obtain baseline neurologic and mental function C. Assess pt for any neurologic abnormalities and report changes to MD D. Discuss with pt the impact of malaise on his or her general sense of well-being and strategies to minimize distress

L-asparaginase *Continued*

Nursing Diagnosis	Defining Characteristics
V. *Alteration in mobility related to soreness at injection site*	V. A. Pt may complain of sore muscle at injection site
VI. *Infection, bleeding, and fatigue related to bone marrow depression*	VI. A. Bone marrow depression is not common B. Mild anemia may occur C. Serious leukopenia and thrombocytopenia are rare
VII. *Potential for sexual dysfunction*	VII. A. Drug is teratogenic

Expected Outcomes	Nursing Interventions
V. A. Pt will not complain of altered mobility due to sore muscles	V. A. Rotate injection sites to decrease potential for soreness B. Utilize standard nursing practice for IM injections
VI. A. Pt will be without s/s of infection, bleeding, or anemia B. Early s/s of infection, bleeding, or anemia will be identified	VI. A. Monitor CBC, platelet count prior to drug administration, as well as s/s of infection, bleeding, or anemia B. Instruct pt in self-assessment of s/s of infection, bleeding, or anemia
VII. A. Pt and significant other will understand need for contraception	VII. A. As appropriate, explore with pt and significant other issues of reproductive and sexual pattern B. Discuss strategies to preserve sexuality and reproductive health (e.g., sperm banking, contraception)

Leucovorin calcium
(Folinic acid, Citrovorum factor)

Class: Water-soluble vitamin in the folate group (folinic acid)

MECHANISM OF ACTION

Acts as an antidote for methotrexate and other folic acid antagonists. Circumvents the biochemical block of the enzyme inhibitors (e.g., dihydrofolate reductase [DHFR]) to permit DNA and RNA synthesis. Used as a potentiator of 5-FU, causes 5-FU to bind more tightly to thymidylate synthetase.

METABOLISM

Metabolized primarily in the liver; 50% of the single dose is excreted in 6 hours in the urine (80–90% of dose) and stool (8% of dose).

DOSAGE/RANGE

Dose of drug and duration of rescue is dependent on serum methotrexate levels.

MTX Level	*Leucovorin*
$< 5.0(10)^{-7}$M	10 mg/m^2 every 6 hours
$5(10){-}7$M to $5(10)^{-6}$M	30–40 mg/m^2 every 6 hours
$> 5(10)^{-6}$M	100 mg/m^2 every 3–6 hours

Drug combinations/dosages are under investigation. The following are sample doses.

5-FU 370 mg/m^2/day for 5 days continuous infusion. Leucovorin 500 mg/m^2/day continuous infusion starting 24 hours before 5-FU and continuing until 12 hours after.

5-FU 600 mg/m^2 plus leucovorin 500 mg/m^2 weekly for 6 weeks

5-FU 350–500 mg/m^2 IVB over 2 hours with leucovorin 350–500 mg/m^2 IVP midway during infusion weekly for 6 weeks

5-FU 500 mg/m^2 qd × 5 plus leucovorin 200 mg/m^2 qd × 5

DRUG PREPARATION

Drug is supplied in ampules or vials. Reconstitute vials with sterile water for injection. Dilute reconstituted vials or ampules further with D$_5$W or normal saline.

DRUG ADMINISTRATION

Administer 24 hours after first methotrexate dose is begun. Dose every 6 hours for up to 12 doses.

First dose is given IV: others can be administered orally or IM.

IV doses are given via bolus over 15 minutes.

Doses must be given *exactly on time* in order to rescue normal cells from methotrexate toxicity.

SPECIAL CONSIDERATIONS

It is imperative that the patient receive the leucovorin on schedule to avoid fatal methotrexate toxicity. Notify the physician if the patient is unable to take the dose orally, as it must then be given IV.

Usually free of side effects but allergic reaction and local pain may occur.

Drug metabolite may accumulate in CSF, thus decreasing effectiveness of intrathecal methotrexate.

Leucovorin calcium

Nursing Diagnosis	Defining Characteristics
I. *Potential for injury related to* A. Allergic reaction	I. A. Allergic sensitization has been reported: facial flushing, itching
B. Drug interaction	B. Leucovorin in large amounts may counteract the antiepileptic effects of phenobarbital, phenytoin, and pyrimidine
II. *Altered nutrition, less than body requirements related to nausea and vomiting*	II. A. Oral leucovorin rarely causes nausea or vomiting

Expected Outcomes	Nursing Interventions
I. A. 1. Pt will be without an allergic reaction 2. If allergic reaction occurs, it will be minimized B. Pt will maintain baseline neurological status	I. A. 1. Monitor pt for s/s of allergic reaction 2. Diphenhydramine is effective for relieving symptoms of allergic reaction B. 1. Monitor pt for symptoms of increased seizure activity (if on antiepileptic drugs) 2. Monitor antiepileptic drug levels
II. A. Pt will be without nausea and vomiting	II. A. Administer oral leucovorin with antacids or milk

Melphalan
(Alkeran, L-PAM, Phenylalanine Mustard, L-sarcolysin)

Class: Alkylating agent

MECHANISM OF ACTION

Prevents cell replication by causing breaks and cross-linkages in DNA strands, with subsequent miscoding and breakage. Is cell cycle phase-nonspecific. Drug is derivative of nitrogen mustard.

METABOLISM

Variable bioavailability after oral administration, especially if taken with food. Therefore, dose is titrated to WBC count; 20–50% of drug is excreted in feces over 6 days, 50% excreted in urine within 24 hours. After IV administration, parent compound disappears from plasma, with a half-life of about 2 hours.

DOSAGE/RANGE

6 mg/m^2 orally daily × 5 days every 6 weeks for myeloma

or

0.1 mg/kg orally × 2–3 weeks, then maintenance of 2–4 mg daily when bone marrow has recovered
8 mg/m^2 IV daily × 5 days (experimental)

DRUG PREPARATION

Oral: available in 2-mg tablets.

IV: dilute reconstituted vial in D_5W. Administer over 30–45 minutes.

DRUG ADMINISTRATION

Serious hypersensitivity reactions reported with IV.

Take oral preparation on an empty stomach.

IV infusion should be given in 100–150 ml of D_5W or NS over 15–30 minutes.

SPECIAL CONSIDERATIONS

Nadir 14–21 days after treatment.

Increased risk of nephrotoxicity when given with cyclosporine.

Doses used in bone marrow transplant are 140–200 mg/m^2.

Drug is used experimentally in regional perfusion.

Drug dose reduction recommended in patients with renal compromise.

Drug activity enhanced with concurrent administration of misonidazol (investigational).

Melphalan

Nursing Diagnosis	Defining Characteristics
I. *Infection and bleeding related to bone marrow depression*	I. A. Bone marrow depression may be pronounced B. Leukopenia and thrombocytopenia 14–21 days after intermittent dosing schedules C. May be delayed in onset and cumulative, with nadir extended to 5–6 weeks D. Combined immunosuppression from disease (i.e., multiple myeloma) and drug may prolong vulnerability to infection E. Thrombocytopenia may be persistent
II. *Altered nutrition, less than body requirements related to* A. Nausea and vomiting	II. A. Mild at low, continuous dosing; severe following high doses
B. Anorexia	B. Occurs rarely
C. Stomatitis	C. Infrequent occurrence (rare)
III. *Impaired skin integrity related to alopecia, maculopapular rash, urticaria*	III. A. Alopecia is minimal, if it occurs at all B. Maculopapular rash and urticaria are infrequent

Expected Outcomes	**Nursing Interventions**
I. A. Pt will be without s/s of infection or bleeding B. Early s/s of infection or bleeding will be identified early	I. A. Monitor CBC, platelets prior to drug administration, and assess for s/s of infection or bleeding B. Hold drug if WBC < 3000/mm^3 or platelet count < 100,000/mm^3; discuss with MD C. Teach pt self-assessment techniques and self-care measures to minimize risk of infection and bleeding

II. A. 1. Pt will be without nausea and vomiting
     2. Nausea and vomiting, if they occur, will be minimal
 	
B. Pt will maintain baseline weight ± 5%
 	
C. Oral mucous membrane will remain intact and without infection
	II. A. 1. Administer drug (oral) on empty stomach
	     2. Premedicate with antiemetic (oral) 1 hr before oral dose
	     3. Use aggressive antiemetic regimen for IV Alkeran
	B. 1. Encourage small, frequent feedings of favorite foods, especially high-calorie, high-protein foods
	     2. Encourage use of spices
	     3. Weekly weights
	C. 1. Teach pt oral assessment
	     2. Assess oral mucosa prior to drug administration
	     3. Encourage pt to report (early) stomatitis

III. A. Pt will develop strategy to manage distress associated with skin side effects	III. A. Assess skin integrity and presence of rash, urticaria, alopecia prior to dosing B. Assess impact of these alterations on pt and develop plan to manage symptom distress

Melphalan *Continued*

Nursing Diagnosis	Defining Characteristics
IV. *Potential for impaired gas exchange related to pulmonary toxicity*	IV. A. Rare but may occur, especially with continued chronic dosing B. Bronchopulmonary dysplasia and pulmonary fibrosis
V. *Potential for injury related to* A. Second malignancy	V. A. 1. Acute myelogenous and myelomonocytic leukemias may occur after continuous long-term dosing 2. Especially in pts with ovarian cancer and multiple myeloma 3. Heralded by preleukemic pancytopenia of several weeks' duration 4. Chromosomal abnormalities characteristic of acute leukemia
B. Drug infiltration when given IV	B. Painful burning can occur
C. Anaphylaxis and hypersensitivity reactions	C. Severe hypersensitivity reactions can occur with IV administration, including diaphoresis, hypotension, and cardiac arrest

Expected Outcomes	Nursing Interventions
IV. A. Early s/s of pulmonary toxicity will be identified	IV. A. Assess pulmonary status for s/s of pulmonary dysfunction B. Assess lung sounds prior to dosing C. Instruct pt to report cough or dyspnea D. Discuss pulmonary function studies to be performed periodically with MD
V. A. Malignancy, if it occurs, will be identified early	V. A. Pts receiving prolonged continuous therapy should be closely followed during and after treatment
B. Drug infiltration will not occur	B. Drug administration technique should be meticulous
C. 1. Hypersensitivity reactions will be detected early 2. Airway will ba patent 3. BP will remain within 20 mmHg of baseline 4. Anaphylaxis, if it occurs, will be detected early	C. 1. Review standing orders for management of pt in anaphylaxis and identify location of anaphylaxis kit containing epinephrine 1:1000, hydrocortisone sodium succinate (SoluCortef), diphenhydramine HCl (Benadryl), Aminophyline, and others 2. Prior to drug administration, obtain baseline vital signs and record mental status 3. Administer drug slowly, diluted as per MD order

Melphalan   *Continued*

Nursing Diagnosis	Defining Characteristics
C. Anaphylaxis and hypersensitivity reactions	

Expected Outcomes	**Nursing Interventions**
	4. Observe for following s/s, usually occurring within first 15 mins of infusion
	a. *Subjective*
	(1) generalized itching
	(2) nausea
	(3) chest tightness
	(4) crampy abdominal pain
	(5) difficulty speaking
	(6) anxiety
	(7) agitation
	(8) sense of impending doom
	(9) uneasiness
	(10) desire to urinate/defecate
	(11) dizziness
	(12) chills
	b. *Objective*
	(1) flushed appearance (angioedema of face, neck, eyelids, hands, feet)
	(2) localized or generalized urticaria
	(3) respiratory distress ± wheezing
	(4) hypotension
	(5) cyanosis
	5. For generalized allergic reaction, stop infusion and notify MD
	6. Place pt in supine position to promote perfusion of visceral organs
	7. Monitor vital signs
	8. Provide emotional reassurance to pt and family
	9. Maintain patent airway and have CPR equipment ready if needed

Melphalan *Continued*

Nursing Diagnosis	Defining Characteristics
C. Anaphylaxis and hypersensitivity reactions	
VI. *Potential for sexual dysfunction*	VI. A. Potentially mutagenic and teratogenic

Expected Outcomes	**Nursing Interventions**
	10. Document incident 11. Discuss with MD desensitization versus drug discontinuance for further dosing
VI. A. Pt and significant other will understand potential sexual dysfunction	VI. A. Encourage pt to verbalize goals re family and discuss options, such as sperm banking B. As appropriate, discuss or refer for counseling re birth control measures during therapy

6-Mercaptopurine
(Purinethol, 6-MP)

Class: Antimetabolite

MECHANISM OF ACTION

One of two thiopurine antimetabolites (with 6-TG) that are converted to monophosphate nucleotides and inhibit de novo purine synthesis. The nucleotides are also incorporated into DNA. Cell cycle phase-specific (S phase).

METABOLISM

Metabolized by the enzyme xanthine oxidase in the kidney and liver. Because xanthine oxidase is inhibited by allopurinol, concurrent use of the latter necessitates a dose reduction of 6-MP to one-fourth the normal dose. Fifty percent of the drug is excreted in the urine. Plasma half-life: 20–40 minutes.

DOSAGE/RANGE

100 mg/m^2 orally daily × 5 days

Children: 70 mg/m^2 daily for induction, then 40 mg/m^2 daily for maintenance

IV use is investigational.

DRUG PREPARATION

Oral: available in 50 mg tablets.

IV: reconstitute 500-mg vial with sterile water for concentration of 10 mg/ml.

Store IV solution at room temperature; discard after 8 hours.

DRUG ADMINISTRATION

IV use is investigational; consult protocol.

SPECIAL CONSIDERATIONS

Elevated serum glucose levels and elevated serum uric acid levels could be related to the effects of medication.

Patients receiving allopurinol concurrently may require dosage reduction due to xanthine oxidase inhibition.

When given with nondepolarizing muscle relaxants, there is decreased neuromuscular blockade.

When given with warfarin, there is a decreased hypothrombinemic effect.

Reduce dose in cases of hepatic or renal dysfunction.

6-Mercaptopurine

Nursing Diagnosis	Defining Characteristics
I. *Altered nutrition, less than body requirements related to*	I.
A. Nausea and vomiting	A. Uncommon; mild when they occur
B. Anorexia	B. Infrequent; mild
C. Stomatitis	C. Uncommon; appears as white patchy areas similar to thrush
D. Diarrhea	D. Occurs occasionally; mild
E. Hepatotoxicity	E. 1. Reversible cholestatic jaundice may develop after 2–5 months of treatment 2. Hepatic necrosis may develop

Expected Outcomes	**Nursing Interventions**
I. A. 1. Pt will be without nausea and vomiting 2. Nausea and vomiting, if they occur, will be minimal	I. A. 1. Consider premedicating with antiemetics for first dose 2. Encourage small, frequent feedings of cool, bland foods and liquids 3. Assess for symptoms of fluid/electrolyte imbalance if pt's vomiting is significant 4. Monitor I&O, daily weights; check lab results
B. Pt will maintain baseline weight ± 5%	B. 1. Encourage small, frequent feedings of favorite foods, especially high-calorie, high-protein foods 2. Encourage use of spices
C. Oral mucous membranes will remain intact and without infection	C. 1. Teach oral assessment and mouth care regimen 2. Encourage pt to report early stomatitis 3. Provide pain relief measures if indicated
D. Pt will have minimal diarrhea	D. 1. Encourage pt to report onset of diarrhea 2. Administer or teach pt to self-administer antidiarrheal medication 3. Guaiac all stools 4. If diarrhea if protracted, ensure adequate hydration, monitor I&O and electrolytes, and teach hygiene to pt
E. Early hepatotoxicity will be identified	E. 1. Monitor SGOT, SGPT, LDH, alkaline phosphatase, and bilirubin periodically during treatment 2. Notify MD of any elevations 3. Hepatotoxicity may be an indication for discontinuing treatment

6-Mercaptopurine   *Continued*

Nursing Diagnosis	Defining Characteristics
II. *Potential for infection and bleeding related to bone marrow depression*	II. A. Nadir varies from 5 days to 6 weeks after treatment B. Leukopenia more prominent than thrombocytopenia C. Blood counts may continue to fall after therapy is stopped
III. *Potential for impaired skin integrity*	III. A. Skin eruptions, rash may occur

Expected Outcomes	**Nursing Interventions**
II. A. Pt will be without s/s of infection or bleeding B. Early s/s of infection or bleeding will be identified	II. A. Monitor CBC, platelet count prior to drug administration, as well as s/s of infection or bleeding B. Instruct in self-assessment of s/s of infection or bleeding
III. A. Distress related to alterations in skin condition will be minimized	III. A. Advise pt these changes may occur B. Instruct pt in symptomatic care if distress related to skin reactions occurs

Methotrexate
(Amethopterin, Mexate, Folex)

Class: Antimetabolite (folic acid antagonist)

MECHANISM OF ACTION

Blocks the enzyme dihydrofolate reductase (DHFR), which inhibits the conversion of folic acid to tetrahydrofolic acid, resulting in an inhibition of the key precursors of DNA, RNA, and cellular proteins. May synchronize malignant cells in the S phase. At high plasma levels, passive entry of the drug into tumor cells can potentially overcome drug resistance.

METABOLISM

Bound to serum albumin; concurrent use of drugs that displace methotrexate from serum albumin should be avoided. Salicylates, sulfonamides, dilantin, some antibacterials (including tetracycline, chloramphenicol, paraminobenzoic acid), and alcohol should be avoided, as they will delay excretion. Drug is absorbed from gastrointestinal tract and peaks in 1 hour. Plasma half-life is 2 hours; 50–100% of dose is excreted into the systemic circulation, with peak concentration 3–12 hours after administration.

DOSAGE/RANGE

IV: Low, 10–50 mg/m^2

       Medium, 100–500 mg/m^2

       High, 500 mg/m^2 and above, with leucovorin rescue

IT: 10–15 mg/m^2

IM: 25 mg/m^2

DRUG PREPARATION

5-mg, 50-mg, 100-mg, and 200-mg vials are available already reconstituted.

Powder is available in vials without preservative for IT and high-dose administration (reconstitute with preservative-free NS).

DRUG ADMINISTRATION

5–149 mg: slow IVP
150–499 mg: IV drip over 20 minutes
500–1500 mg: infusion per protocol, with leucovorin rescue

SPECIAL CONSIDERATIONS

High doses cross the blood-brain barrier: reconstitute with preservative-free NS.

With high doses ($1–7.5 \text{ gm/m}^2$), urine should be alkalinized both before and after administration, as the drug is a weak acid and can crystallize in the kidneys at an acid pH. Alkalinize with bicarbonate and add to prehydration and posthydration. High doses should be given only under the direction of a qualified oncologist at an institution that can provide rapid serum methotrexate level readings.

Leucovorin rescue must be given *on time* per orders to prevent excessive toxicity and to achieve maximum therapeutic response (see leucovorin calcium table).

Avoid folic acid and its derivatives during methotrexate therapy.

Kidney function must be adequate to excrete drug and avoid excessive toxicity. Check BUN and creatinine before each dose.

Methotrexate

Nursing Diagnosis	Defining Characteristics
I. *Altered nutrition, less than body requirements related to*	I.
A. Nausea and vomiting	A. 1. Nausea and vomiting uncommon with low dose; more common (39%) with high dose 2. May occur during drug administration and last 24–72 hours
B. Stomatitis	B. 1. Common; indication for interruption of therapy 2. Occurs in 3–5 days with high dose, 3–4 weeks with low dose 3. Appears initially at corners of mouth
C. Diarrhea	C. 1. Common; indication for interruption of therapy, as enteritis and intestinal perforation may occur 2. Melena, hematemesis may occur
D. Hepatotoxicity	D. 1. Usually subclinical and reversible but can lead to cirrhosis 2. Increased risk of hepatotoxicity when given with other hepatotoxic agents, like alcohol 3. Transient increase in LFTs with high dose 1–10 days after treatment; pt may become jaundiced
E. Anorexia	E. Mild

Expected Outcomes	**Nursing Interventions**

I. A. 1. Pt will be without nausea and vomiting
      2. Nausea and vomiting, should they occur, will be minimal
	I. A. 1. Premedicate with antiemetics if giving high-dose methotrexate; continue prophylactically for 24 hrs (at least) to prevent nausea and vomiting
	      2. Encourage small, frequent feedings of cool, bland foods and liquids
	      3. Assess for symptoms of fluid and electrolyte imbalance; monitor I&O, daily weights if inpt

B. Oral mucous membranes will remain intact and without infection	B. 1. Assess oral cavity every day
	    2. Teach pt oral assessment and mouth care regimens
	    3. Encourage pt to report early stomatitis
	    4. Provide pain relief measures if indicated
	    5. Explore pt compliance to rescue; discuss ↑ rescue dose

C. Pt will have minimal diarrhea	C. 1. Assess pt for diarrhea; guaiac all stools
	    2. Encourage pt to report onset of diarrhea
	    3. Administer or teach pt to self-administer antidiarrheal medications

D. Early hepatotoxicity will be identified	D. 1. Monitor LFTs prior to drug dose, especially with high-dose methotrexate 2. Assess pt prior to and during treatment for s/s of hepatotoxicity

E. Pt will maintain baseline weight ±5%	E. 1. Encourage small, frequent feedings of favorite foods, especially high-calorie, high-protein foods
	    2. Encourage use of spices
	    3. Daily weights

Methotrexate *Continued*

Nursing Diagnosis	Defining Characteristics
II. *Potential for infection and bleeding related to bone marrow depression*	II. A. Nadir seen 7–9 days after drug administration B. Nadir range: WBC, 4–7 days; platelets, 5–12 days C. Bone marrow depression of pts
III. *Potential for altered urinary elimination related to renal toxicity*	III. A. As an organic acid, methotrexate is insoluble in acid urine B. At doses greater than 1 gm/m^2 (i.e., high dose), drug may precipitate in renal tubules, causing acute tubular necrosis (ATN)
IV. *Potential for impaired gas exchange related to pulmonary toxicity*	IV. A. Pneumothorax (high dose) rare; occurs within first 48 hours after drug administration in pts with pulmonary metastasis B. Allergic pneumonitis (high dose) rare but accompanied by eosinophilia, patchy pulmonary infiltrates, fever, cough, shortness of breath; occurs 1–5 months after initiation of treatment C. Pneumonitis (low dose) symptoms usually disappear within a week, with or without use of steroids; interstitial pneumonitis may be a fatal complication

Expected Outcomes	Nursing Interventions
II. A. Pt will be without s/s of infection or bleeding B. S/s of infection or bleeding will be identified early	II. A. Monitor CBC, platelet count prior to drug administration, as well as s/s of infection or bleeding B. Instruct pt in self-assessment of s/s of infection or bleeding C. Administer leucovorin calcium as ordered D. See care plan for leucovorin calcium
III. A. Pt will maintain normal patterns of urinary elimination B. Renal toxicity will be avoided	III. A. Prehydrate pt with alkaline solution for several hours prior to drug administration B. Maintain high urine output with a urine pH of greater than 7 (hydration fluid may need further alkalinization); dipstick each void C. Record I&O D. Monitor BUN and serum creatinine before, during, and after drug administration; increases in these values may require methotrexate dose reductions or leucovorin dose increases
IV. A. Early s/s of pulmonary toxicity will be identified	IV. A. Assess for s/s of pulmonary dysfunction before each dose and between doses (see "Defining Characteristics") B. Discuss pulmonary function studies to be performed periodically with MD C. Assess lung sounds prior to drug administration D. Instruct pt to report cough or dyspnea

Methotrexate *Continued*

Nursing Diagnosis	Defining Characteristics
V. *Potential for alteration in skin integrity*	V. A. Alopecia and dermatitis are uncommon B. Pruritis and urticaria may occur C. Photosensitivity and sunburn-like rash 1–5 days after treatment; also radiation recall reaction
VI. *Potential for sensory and perceptual alterations*	VI. A. CNS effects: dizziness, malaise, blurred vision B. IT administration may increase CSF pressure C. Brain XRT followed by IV MTX may cause neurological changes
VII. *Potential for alterations in comfort*	VII. A. Sometimes causes back pain during administration

Expected Outcomes	Nursing Interventions
V. A. Pt will verbalize feelings about potential change in body image and identify strategies to cope with them B. Pt will identify strategies to minimize, avoid, or treat body image change	V. A. Assess pt for s/s of hair loss B. Discuss with pt impact of hair loss and strategies to minimize distress C. Instruct pt to avoid sun if possible, to stay covered or wear sunscreen if sun exposure is unavoidable
VI. A. Early s/s of neurological toxicity will be identified	VI. A. Monitor for CNS effects of drug: dizziness, blurred vision, malaise B. Monitor for symptoms of increased CSF pressure: seizures, paresis, headache, nausea and vomiting, brain atrophy, fever C. If IV methotrexate follows brain XRT, monitor for symptoms of increased CSF pressure
VII. A. Pt will report comfort throughout drug administration	VII. A. Monitor pt for back and flank pain; slow infusion rate if it occurs B. Administer analgesics if pain occurs (must avoid ASA-containing products, as they displace methotrexate from serum albumin)

Mitoxantrone
(Novantrone)

Class: Anthracenediones; antitumor antibiotic

MECHANISM OF ACTION

Inhibits both DNA and RNA synthesis regardless of the phase of cell division. Intercalates between base pairs, thus distorting DNA structure. DNA-dependent RNA synthesis and protein synthesis are also inhibited.

METABOLISM

Excreted in both the bile and urine for 24–36 hours as virtually unchanged drug. Mean half-life is 5.8 hours. Peak levels achieved immediately. FDA approved for acute nonlymphocytic leukemia in adults.

DOSAGE/RANGE

10–14 mg/m^2 daily for 1–3 days
10–24 mg/m^2/day (clinical trials; see specific protocol)

DRUG PREPARATION

Available as dark blue solution.

May be diluted in D_5W, NS, or D_5NS.

Solution is chemically stable at room temperature for at least 48 hours.

Intact vials should be stored at room temperature. If refrigerated, a precipitate may form. This precipitate can be redissolved when vial is warmed to room temperature.

DRUG ADMINISTRATION

IV push over 3 minutes through the arm of a freely running infusion.

IV bolus over 5–30 minutes.

SPECIAL CONSIDERATIONS

Nonvesicant. There have been rare reports of tissue necrosis after drug infiltration.

Incompatible with admixtures containing heparin.

Patient may experience blue-green urine for 24 hours after drug administration.

Mitoxantrone

Nursing Diagnosis	Defining Characteristics
I. *Potential for injury related to*	I.

A. Infection	A. 1. Significant bone marrow depression; nadir 9–10 days
	    2. Granulocytopenia is usually the dose-limiting toxicity
	    3. Toxicity may be cumulative

B. Bleeding	B. Thrombocytopenia uncommon but can be severe when it occurs

C. Allergic reactions	C. 1. Hypersensitivity has been reported occasionally
	    2. Hypotension
	    3. Urticaria
	    4. Dyspnea
	    5. Rashes

II. *Nutrition alteration, less than body requirements related to*	II.
A. Nausea and vomiting	A. 1. Typically not severe 2. Occurs in 30% of pts

B. Mucositis	B. 1. More common with prolonged dosing
	    2. Occurs in 5% of pts
	    3. Usually within 1 week of therapy

Expected Outcomes	**Nursing Interventions**
I. A. 1. Pt will be without infection 2. Early s/s of infection and bleeding will be identified	I. A. 1. Monitor WBC, hematocrit, platelets prior to drug administration 2. Drug dosage should be reduced or held for lower-than-normal blood values 3. Instruct pt in self-assessment of s/s of infection
B. 1. Pt will be without s/s of bleeding 2. Bleeding, if it occurs, will be identified and treated early C. Allergic reactions will be detected early	B. Instruct pt in self-assessment of s/s of bleeding C. 1. Prior to drug administration, obtain baseline vital signs 2. Observe for s/s of allergic reaction 3. Subjective s/s: generalized itching, dizziness 4. Objective s/s: flushed appearance (angioedema of face, neck, eyelids, hands, feet), localized or generalized urticaria 5. Document incident 6. Discuss with MD desensitization for future dose versus drug discontinuance
II. A. 1. Pt will be without nausea and vomiting 2. Nausea and vomiting, if they occur, will be minimal	II. A. 1. Premedicate with antiemetic and continue prophylactically × 24 hrs to prevent nausea and vomiting, at least for first treatment 2. Encourage small, frequent feedings of cool, bland foods and liquids
B. Oral mucous membranes will remain intact and without infection	B. 1. Teach pt oral assessment and oral hygiene regimen 2. Encourage pt to report early stomatitis

Mitoxantrone *Continued*

Nursing Diagnosis	Defining Characteristics
III. *Potential for impaired skin integrity related to* A. Alopecia	III. A. 1. Mild to moderate 2. Occurs in 20% of pts
B. Extravasation	B. 1. Not a vesicant 2. Stains skin blue, without ulcers 3. Rare reports of tissue necrosis following extravasation
IV. *Potential for alteration in cardiac output*	IV. A. CHF B. Decreased left ventricular ejection fraction occurs in about 3% of pts C. Increased cardiotoxicity with cumulative dose greater than 180 mg/m^2 D. Cumulative lifetime dose must be reduced if pt has had previous anthracycline therapy

Expected Outcomes	**Nursing Interventions**

III. A. 1. Pt will verbalize feelings regarding hair loss
   2. Pt will identify strategies to cope with change in body image
	III. A. 1. Discuss with pt impact of hair loss
	   2. Suggest wig as appropriate prior to actual hair loss
	   3. Explore with pt response to actual hair loss and plan strategies to minimize distress, (e.g., wig, scarf, cap)

B. 1. Skin discomfort will be minimized
   2. Skin will remain intact
   3. Pt will verbalize feelings re skin changes
	B. 1. Use careful technique during venipuncture
	   2. Administer drug through freely flowing IV, constantly monitoring IV site and pt response
	   3. Teach pt to assess site and notify provider if condition worsens
	   4. Arrange next clinic visit for assessment of site depending on drug, amount infiltrated, extent of potential injury, and pt variables
	   5. Document in pt's record as per institutional policy and procedure

IV. A. Early s/s of cardiomyopathy will be identified	IV. A. Assess for s/s of cardiomyopathy
	   B. Assess quality and regularity of heartbeat
	   C. Baseline EKG
	   D. Instruct pt to report dyspnea, shortness of breath, swelling of extremities, orthopnea
	   E. Discuss frequency of gated blood pool scan with MD

Mitoxantrone *Continued*

Nursing Diagnosis	Defining Characteristics
V. *Alteration in metabolic pattern*	V. A. In leukemia pts, rapid tumor lysis may occur, with resultant hyperuricemia
VI. *Potential for anxiety*	VI. A. Urine will be green/blue for 24 hrs B. Sclera may become discolored blue
VII. *Potential for sexual dysfunction*	VII. A. Drug is mutagenic and teratogenic

Expected Outcomes	Nursing Interventions
V. A. Hyperuricemia will be identified early	V. A. Hydrate pt B. Alkalinize urine C. Administer allopurinol as per MD order D. Evaluate the effects of allopurinol by monitoring uric acid levels E. Monitor blood values of electrolytes, BUN, and creatinine
VI. A. Pt will verbalize understanding of physiological changes expected with treatment	VI. A. Explain to pt changes that may occur with therapy and that they are only temporary
VII. A. Pt and significant other will understand the need for contraception	VII. A. As appropriate, explore with pt and significant other issues of reproductive and sexuality pattern and impact chemotherapy may have B. Discuss strategies to preserve sexual and reproductive health (e.g., sperm banking, contraception)

Paclitaxel
(Taxol)

Class: Mitotic inhibitor (spindle poison)

MECHANISM OF ACTION

Promotes early microtubule assembly; prevents depolymerization, bringing about cell arrest.

METABOLISM

Extensively protein bound, resulting in an initial sharp decline in serum levels; metabolized by the liver. Metabolites excreted in bile.

DOSAGE/RANGE

Previously untreated ovarian cancer: 135 mg/m^2 IV over 24 hours, followed by cisplatin 75 mg/m^2 every 3 weeks.

Previously treated ovarian cancer: 135–175 mg/m^2 IV over 3 hours every 3 weeks.

Adjuvant node positive breast cancer: 175 mg/m^2 IV over 3 hours, every 3 weeks, for 4 courses administered sequentially to doxorubicin-containing combination chemotherapy.

Metastatic breast cancer overexpressing HER2 protein: 175 mg/m^2 IV over 3 hours, every 3 weeks in combination with trastuzumab.

Metastatic breast cancer, after failure of initial therapy or relapse within 6 months of adjuvant therapy: 175 mg/m^2 IV over 3 hours every 3 weeks.

Non-small-cell lung cancer (NSCLC), not candidate for potentially curative surgery and/or XRT: 135 mg/m^2 IV over 24 hours, followed by cisplatin 75 mg/m^2 repeated every 3 weeks.

Second line AIDS-related Kaposi's Sarcoma: 135 mg/m^2 IV over 3 hours, repeated every 3 weeks or 100 mg/m^2 IV over 3 hours, repeated every 2 weeks (dose intensity of 45–50 mg/m^2 per week).

Other regimes used/being studied/reported: Advanced or metastatic NSCLC Phase II study of weekly paclitaxel 50 mg/m^2 IV over 1 hour in combination with carboplatin AUC 2 with concurrent XRT, and after completion of XRT, paclitaxel 200 mg/m^2 and carboplatin AUC 6 q 3 weeks × 2 cycles; studies in other tumor types (bladder, small cell lung, head and neck cancers).

DRUG PREPARATION

Taxol is poorly soluble in water, so it is formulated using Cremaphor EL (polyoxyethylated castor oil) and dehydrated alcohol. Dilute in 5% dextrose or 0.9% sodium chloride.

DRUG ADMINISTRATION

IV as 3-hour infusion or 24-hour continuous infusion, repeated every 21 days.

Glass or polyolefin containers and polyethylene-lined nitroglycerine tubing *must be used. Do not use* polyvinyl chloride plastic, as diethylhexlphthalate leaches into drug solution.

Use 0.22-micron in-line filter.

(continued)

(Paclitaxel continued)

SPECIAL CONSIDERATIONS

Premedicate with steroid, H_2 blocker, diphenhydramine to prevent hypersensitivity reaction.

Reversal of multidrug resistance experimentally successful with quinidine, cyclosporin A, quinine, or verapamil.

Has radiosensitizing effects.

Hypersensitivity reactions occur in 10% of patients, and cardiac arrythmias can occur; keep resuscitation equipment nearby.

Monitor vital signs every 15 minutes for 1 hour and then every hour if no adverse effects occur.

Do not give drug as a bolus, as it may cause bronchospasm and hypotension.

Phlebitis may occur rarely.

Drug is embryofetal toxic; benefit should outweigh risk if drug is used during pregnancy.

Breast-feeding should be avoided, as drug may be excreted in breast milk.

Contraindicated in patients with hypersensitivity to paclitaxel or other drugs formulated in Cremaphor EL. However, there are reports of rechallenge following multiple high doses of corticosteroids.

Contraindicated in patients with baseline absolute neutrophil count < 1500 cells/mm^3, and < 1000 cells/mm^3 in AIDS-related Kaposi's Sarcoma patients.

Drug may interact with ketoconazole, resulting in decreased paclitaxel metabolism; monitor patient closely.

If severe neuropathy develops, drug dose should be reduced 20%.

Paclitaxel

Nursing Diagnosis	Defining Characteristics
I. *Potential for injury related to hypersensitivity reactions*	I. A. 10% of pts experience anaphylaxis B. S/s include tachycardia, wheezing, hypotension, facial edema, supraventricular tachycardia with hypotension and chest pain (1–2%)

Expected Outcomes	**Nursing Interventions**
I. A. Early s/s of hypersensitivity reactions will be identified	I. A. Review standing orders for management of hypersensitivity reactions and identify location of anaphylaxis kit containing epinephrine 1:1000, hydrocortisone sodium succinate (SoluCortef), diphenhydramine HCl (Benadryl), Aminophylline, and other medications

B. Prior to drug administration, obtain baseline vital signs and record mental status assessment

C. Administer or teach pt to self-administer (as ordered) the following:
1. Dexamethasone 20-mg IV or po 12–14 hrs and 6–7 hrs prior to paclitaxel administration
2. Diphenhydramine 50-mg IV 30 mins prior to chemotherapy
3. Ranitidine 50-mg IV or cimetidine 300 mg IV or other H_2 blocker 30 mins prior to chemotherapy

D. Assess pt for at least 30 mins after drug is given for s/s of a reaction

E. Teach pt to report any hypersensitivity reactions or unusual symptoms

F. Observe for the following s/s during infusion, usually occurring within first 15 mins of start of infusion:
1. *Subjective*
   a. Generalized itching
   b. Nausea
   c. Chest tightness
   d. Crampy abdominal pain
   e. Difficulty speaking
   f. Anxiety
   g. Agitation
   h. Sense of impending doom
   i. Uneasiness
   j. Desire to urinate or defecate
   k. Dizziness
   l. Chills

Paclitaxel *Continued*

Nursing Diagnosis	Defining Characteristics
I. *Potential for injury related to hypersensitivity reactions*	
II. *Potential alteration in cardiac output*	II. A. Sinus bradycardia occurs in 29% of pts up to 8 hrs after drug infusion B. Ventricular tachycardia rare
III. *Infection and bleeding related to bone marrow depression*	III. A. Neutropenia may be severe; nadir 7–10 days after dose, with recovery in 1 week B. Neutropenia is dose dependent, with severe neutropenia (ANC <500 cells/mm^3) occurring in 47–67% of pts C. Pts with prior XRT are at risk D. Anemia occurs frequently, but thrombocytopenia is uncommon

Expected Outcomes	Nursing Interventions
	2. *Objective* a. Flushed appearance (angioedema of face, lips, neck, eyelids, hands) b. Localized or generalized urticaria c. Respiratory distress ±wheezing d. Hypotension e. Cyanosis G. If reaction occurs, stop infusion and notify MD H. Place pt in supine position to promote perfusion of visceral organs I. Monitor vital signs until stable J. Provide emotional support to pt and family K. Maintain patent airway and have equipment for CPR close by L. Document incident and pt response to treatment M. Discuss with MD desensitization and increased premedication for future treatments
II. A. Cardiac arrhythmias will be identified early B. BP will remain within normal limits	II. A. Assess baseline cardiac status, including apical pulse, and note rate and rhythm; repeat every 15 mins for 1 hr then every hour if stable B. Notify MD if abnormalities occur, and prepare to stabilize pt C. Teach pt to report any discomfort, dizziness, weakness, chest pain
III. A. Pt will be without s/s of infection or bleeding B. Early s/s of infection or bleeding will be identified	III. A. Monitor CBC, platelet count prior to drug administration and postchemotherapy; assess for s/s of infection or bleeding B. Teach pt self-assessment of s/s of infection or bleeding and how to seek medical advice/care C. Teach pt self-administration of granulocyte colony-stimulating factor (G-CSF) as ordered

Paclitaxel *Continued*

Nursing Diagnosis	Defining Characteristics
IV. *Potential for sensory/ perceptual alterations*	IV. A. Peripheral neuropathy may occur within 24 hrs of high-dose therapy (burning pain in feet, hyperesthesias, numbness, periorbital numbness, decreased deep tendon reflexes); severity is dose dependent B. Mild paresthesias most common (62%) C. Symptoms improve within months of drug discontinuance
V. *Alteration in skin integrity related to alopecia*	V. A. Complete alopecia occurs in most pts B. Reversible
VI. *Alteration in nutrition, less than body requirements related to* A. Nausea and vomiting	VI. A. Nausea and vomiting are usually mild and preventable with antiemetics; incidence is 59%
B. Diarrhea	B. Mild, with 43% incidence

Expected Outcomes	**Nursing Interventions**
IV. A. Early s/s of neurological toxicity will be identified B. Function will be maintained	IV. A. Assess baseline neuromuscular function and, prior to drug infusion, especially presence of paresthesias B. Teach pt to report any changes in sensation or function C. Discuss alterations with MD D. Identify strategies to promote comfort and safety
V. A. Pt will verbalize feelings re hair loss and strategies to cope with change in body image	V. A. 1. Discuss potential impact of hair loss prior to drug administration, coping strategies, and plan to minimize body image distortion (e.g., wig, scarf, cap) 2. Assess pt for s/s of hair loss 3. Assess pt's response and use of coping strategies
VI. A. 1. Pt will be without nausea and vomiting 2. Nausea and vomiting, if they occur, will be mild 3. Pt will maintain weight within 5% of baseline B. Pt will have minimal diarrhea	VI. A. 1. Premedicate with antiemetics prior to drug administration and postchemotherapy 2. Encourage small, frequent feedings of cool, bland foods and liquids 3. Assess for symptoms of fluid/electrolyte imbalance if pt has severe nausea and vomiting 4. Monitor I&O, daily weights, lab electrolyte values B. 1. Encourage pt to report onset of diarrhea 2. Administer or teach pt to self-administer antidiarrheal medication

Paclitaxel *Continued*

Nursing Diagnosis	Defining Characteristics
C. Mucositis	C. Mild, with 39% incidence
D. Dysgeusia	D. Occurs rarely
E. Hepatotoxicity	E. Mild increase in liver function studies may occur
VII. *Alteration in comfort related to flu-like syndrome*	VII. A. Occurs rarely and may include arthralgias, myalgias, fever, rash, headache, and fatigue

Expected Outcomes	**Nursing Interventions**
C. Oral mucous membranes will remain infection-free	C. 1. Assess baseline oral mucous membranes 2. Teach pt oral assessment and mouth care and to report any alterations
D. Taste distortions will be minimized	D. 1. Assess presence of taste distortions and ask pt to identify abnormal taste responses to specific foods 2. Discuss alternative foods that do not cause dysgeusia 3. Discuss use of condiments that may minimize dysgeusia (e.g., Crazy Jane salt and pepper) 4. Refer to nutritionist/dietitian as appropriate
E. Hepatic dysfunction will be identified early	E. 1. Assess liver function studies prior to drug administration and periodically during treatment 2. Dose modification necessary for severe hepatic dysfunction (see "Special Considerations")
VII. A. Pt will report early s/s of flu-like syndrome	VII. A. Teach pt about the potential for flu-like syndrome and how to distinguish from actual infection B. Instruct pt to report symptoms C. Teach pt self-care measures to minimize symptoms

Pentostatin
(2'-deoxycofomycin, DCF)

Class: Antitumor antibiotic (investigational)

MECHANISM OF ACTION

Cell cycle phase-nonspecific. A potent inhibitor of adenosine deaminase. Interferes with DNA replication and disrupts RNA processing. It has potent lymphocytotoxic properties. The major mechanism of action is not yet clearly understood.

METABOLISM

The majority of pentostatin is excreted from the body via urine as unchanged drug. The mean halflife is 4.9–6.2 hours.

Clinical trials have shown a relationship between pentostatin's complete excretion and the patient's renal function. Patients with creatinine clearance ≤ 50 ml/min should *not* receive this agent.

DOSAGE/RANGE

Drug is undergoing clinical trials; consult individual protocol for specific dosages.

DRUG PREPARATION

This drug is supplied by the National Cancer Institute.

Available as a white powder.

Reconstitute with sodium chloride injection.

This solution is chemically stable at room temperature for at least 72 hours, but since it lacks bacteriostatic preservatives, discard the solution after 8 hours.

DRUG ADMINISTRATION

Drug is a vesicant. Administer IV push over 5 minutes through the sidearm of a freely running IV.

SPECIAL CONSIDERATIONS

Drug is a vesicant.

Dose-limiting toxicities involve renal and neurotoxicities.

Requires adequate renal function.

Enhanced toxicity when allopurinol is administered concurrently. *Avoid concurrent use.*

Severe, potentially fatal pulmonary toxicity when drug is administered with fludarabine. *Avoid concurrent use.*

Pentostatin

Nursing Diagnosis	Defining Characteristics
I. *Potential for infection and bleeding related to bone marrow depression*	I. A. Severe/profound leukopenia and thrombocytopenia B. Mild anemia
II. *Potential for altered urinary elimination related to nephrotoxicity*	II. A. Renal insufficiency—mild, increased BUN and creatinine common—reversible B. May include hyperuricemia if hydration, allopurinol are inadequate or if tumor lysis is acute
III. *Altered nutrition, less than body requirements related to* A. Nausea and vomiting	III. A. Nausea and vomiting may be mild to severe and seen in at least two-thirds of pts
B. Hepatic dysfunction	B. Hepatitis is rare but may occur; disturbances in liver functions, (i.e., mild SGOT)

IV. *Potential for mental status changes*	IV. A. Neurotoxicity varies from lethargy to somnolence to coma
	    B. Occurs in 60% of cases
	    C. Begins several days after pentostatin infusion and may last for up to 3 weeks

Expected Outcomes	Nursing Interventions
I. A. Pt will be without s/s of infection or bleeding B. Early s/s of infection or bleeding will be identified	I. A. Monitor CBC, platelet count prior to drug administration, as well as s/s of infection or bleeding B. Instruct pt in self-assessment of s/s of infection or bleeding C. Dose reduction often necessary (35–50%) with compromised bone marrow function D. Transfuse with platelets, red cells per MD order
II. A. Pt will be without s/s of nephrotoxicity	II. A. Monitor BUN and creatinine prior to drug dose, as drug is excreted in urine B. Provide or instruct pt in hydration of at least 3 liters of fluid/day C. Monitor I&O D. Hold drug if renal functions are elevated
III. A. 1. Pt will be without nausea and vomiting 2. Nausea and vomiting, if they occur, will be minimal B. Hepatic dysfunction will be identified early	III. A. 1. Premedicate with antiemetics and continue prophylactically × 24 hrs to prevent nausea and vomiting 2. Encourage small, frequent feedings of cool, bland foods and liquids B. 1. Monitor LFTs, especially SGOT 2. Notify MD of any elevations
IV. A. Neurotoxicity will be identified early	IV. A. Teach pt about the potential for neurological reactions and to report any unusual symptoms B. Obtain baseline neurological and mental function C. Assess pt for any neurological abnormalities and report changes to MD

Pentostatin *Continued*

Nursing Diagnosis	Defining Characteristics
IV. *Potential for mental status changes*	
V. *Potential for impaired gas exchange related to pulmonary toxicity*	V. A. Infiltrates and nodules may occur in pts with prior history of receiving bleomycin or lung irradiation
VI. *Potential for sensory/ perceptual alterations*	VI. A. Severe yet reversible conjunctivitis B. Responds to steroid eyedrops
VII. *Alteration in skin integrity related to extravasation*	VII. A. Pentostatin is a potent vesicant B. Vesicants cause erythema, burning, tissue necrosis, tissue sloughing

Expected Outcomes	Nursing Interventions
	D. Concomitant psychotropic drugs may exacerbate s/s
V. A. Early s/s of pulmonary toxicity will be identified	V. A. Obtain baseline pulmonary function B. Assess for s/s of pulmonary dysfunction (i.e., lung sounds) C. Discuss with MD pulmonary function studies to be performed periodically D. Instruct pt to report cough or dyspnea
VI. A. Conjunctivitis will be prevented (or at least identified early)	VI. A. Obtain baseline ophthalmic assessment B. Teach pt of the potential of ophthalmic reactions and to report any unusual symptoms C. Administer steroid eyedrops during drug administration

VII.   A. Extravasation, if it occurs, is detected early, with early intervention
B. Skin and underlying tissue damage is minimized
	VII. A. Use careful technique during venipuncture
	B. Administer vesicant through freely flowing IV, constantly monitoring IV site and pt response
	C. Nurse should be *thoroughly* familiar with institutional policy and procedure for administration of a vesicant agent
	D. If vesicant drug is administered as a continuous infusion, drug must be given through a patent central line
	E. If extravasation is suspected:
	  1. Stop drug being administered
	  2. Aspirate any residual drug and blood from IV tubing, IV catheter/needle, and IV site if possible

Pentostatin *Continued*

Nursing Diagnosis	Defining Characteristics
VII. *Alteration in skin integrity related to extravasation*	

Expected Outcomes	Nursing Interventions
	3. *If antidote exists,* instill antidote into area of apparent infiltration as per MD order and institutional policy and procedure
	4. Apply cold or topical medication as per MD order and institutional policy and procedure
	F. Assess site regularly for pain, progression of erythema, induration, and evidence of necrosis
	G. When in doubt about whether drug is infiltrating, *treat as an infiltration*
	H. Teach pt to assess site and notify MD if condition worsens
	I. Arrange next clinic visit for assessment of site depending on drug, amount infiltrated, extent of potential injury, and pt variables
	J. Document in pt's record as per institutional policy and procedure

Polifeprosan 20 with carmustine (BCNU) implant
(Gliadel™)

Class: Alkylating agent

MECHANISM OF ACTION

Wafer (copolymer) containing carmustine is implanted in the surgical
cavity created when brain tumor is resected. In water, the anhy-
dride bonds of the wafer are hydrolyzed, releasing the carmustine
into the surgical cavity. The carmustine diffuses into the sur-
rounding brain tissue, reaching any residual tumor cells, and causing cell death by alkylating DNA and RNA.

METABOLISM

Unknown. Wafer is biogradable in brain tissue, with a variable rate.
More than 70% of the copolymer degrades by 3 weeks. In some
patients, wafer fragments remained up to 232 days after implan-
tation, with almost all drug gone.

DOSAGE/RANGE

Each wafer contains 7.7 mg of carmustine, and the recommended
dose is 8 wafers, or a total dose of 61.6 mg of carmustine.

DRUG PREPARATION

Drug must be stored at or below $-20°$ C ($-4°$ F) until time of use. Unopened foil packages can stay at room temperature for a maximum of 6 hours at a time. The manufacturer recommends that the treatment box be removed from the freezer and taken to the operating room just prior to surgery. The box and pouches should be opened just before the surgeon is ready to implant the wafers. Open the sealed treatment box and remove double foil packages, handling the unsterile outer foil packet by the crimped edge *very carefully* to prevent damage to the wafers. See product information for opening the inner foil pouch and removing the wafer with sterile technique. Chemotherapy precautions should be used to limit exposure to the chemotherapy: surgical instruments used to remove and implant the wafers should be kept separate from other instruments and sterile fields, and should be cleaned after the procedure according to hospital chemotherapy procedure; all personnel handling the inner foil pouches containing the wafers, or the wafers, should wear double gloves, which, along with unused wafers or fragments, inner foil packages, opened outer foil package, and gloves, should be disposed of as chemotherapeutic waste.

DRUG ADMINISTRATION

Neurosurgeon places 8 wafers into surgical resection cavity if size and shape appropriate; wafers are placed contiguously or with slight overlapping. Wafer may be broken into 2 pieces *only* if needed.

(continued)

(Polifeprosan 20 continued)

DRUG INTERACTIONS

Unknown but unlikely as drug is probably not systemically absorbed.

LAB EFFECTS/INTERFERENCE

Unknown, but unlikely.

SPECIAL CONSIDERATIONS

Indicated for use as an adjunct to surgery to prolong survival in patients with recurrent glioblastoma multiforme for whom surgical resection is indicated.

Manufacturer reports that in a study of 222 patients with recurrent glioma who failed initial surgery and radiotherapy, 6-month survival rate after surgery increased from 47% (placebo) to 60%, and in patients with glioblastoma multiforme. Six-month survival for patients receiving placebo was 36% vs. 56% for patients receiving polifeprosan 20 with carmustine implant.

Patients require close monitoring for complications of craniotomy, as intracerebral mass effect has occurred that does not respond to corticosteroid treatment, and in one case, resulted in brain herniation.

Studies have not been conducted during pregnancy or in nursing mothers. Carmustine is a known teratogen and is embryotoxic. Use during pregnancy should be avoided, and mothers should stop nursing during use of the drug.

Polifeprosan 20

Nursing Diagnosis	Defining Characteristics
I. *Potential sensory/ perceptual alterations related to seizures, brain edema, mental status changes*	I. A. Incidence of new or worsened seizures was 19% in both the group receiving the implant and those receiving the placebo. Seizures were mild to moderate in severity. In pts with new or worsened seizures postoperatively, the group receiving the implant had a 56% incidence, with median time to first new or worsened seizure of 3.5 days, versus placebo incidence of 9%, and median time to first new or worsened seizure of 61 days. Incidence of brain edema was 4%, and there were cases of intracerebral mass effect that did not respond to corticosteroids B. Other nervous system effects: hydrocephalus (3%), depression (3%), abnormal thinking (2%), ataxia (2%), dizziness (2%), insomnia (2%), visual field defect (2%), eye pain (1%), monoplegia (2%), coma (1%), amnesia (1%), diplopia (1%), and paranoid reaction (1%) C. Rarely (< 1%), cerebral infarct or hemorrhage may occur
II. *Potential for infection related to healing abnormalities*	II. A. 1. Most abnormalities were mild to moderate, occurred in 14% of pts, and included: cerebrospinal leaks, subdural fluid collections, subgaleal or wound effusions and breakdown 2. The incidence of intracranial infection (e.g., meningitis or abscess) was 4% B. Incidence of deep wound infection was 6% (same as placebo) and included infection of subgaleal space, bone, meninges, and brain tissue

Expected Outcomes	Nursing Interventions
I. A. Early s/s of increased ICP or CNS changes will be detected and managed	I. A. Monitor neurovital signs closely postoperatively, and notify MD of any abnormalities B. Expect pt to be taken to surgery for removal of the wafer or remnants if increased ICP, or a mass effect is suspected that is unresponsive to corticosteroids C. Assess baseline mental status and regularly postoperatively; validate any changes with family members, report any changes immediately to MD, and continue to monitor neurovital signs closely
II. A. Pt will be without s/s of infection B. If infection develops, s/s will be identified early and managed	II. A. Using aseptic technique, assess postoperative wound dressing immediately after surgery and regularly thereafter B. Assess systematically for s/s of infection or wound breakdown C. If s/s infection or wound breakdown, discuss management and antimicrobial therapy with MD

Polifeprosan 20 *Continued*

Nursing Diagnosis	Defining Characteristics
III. *Alteration in nutrition, less than body requirements related to GI side effects, electrolyte abnormalities*	III. A. Rarely, GI disturbances occurred: diarrhea (2%), constipation (2%), dysphagia (1%), gastrointestinal hemorrhage (1%), fecal incontinence (1%) B. Hyponatremia (3%), hypokalemia (1%), and hyperglycemia (3%) also occurred
IV. *Alteration in circulation, potential, related to changes in blood pressure*	IV. A. Hypertension occurred in 3% of pts, and hypotension in 1%
V. *Alteration in comfort related to edema, pain, asthenia*	V. A. The following occur rarely: peripheral edema (2%), neck pain (2%), rash (2%), back pain (1%), asthenia (1%), chest pain (1%)

Expected Outcomes	Nursing Interventions
III. A. Pt will maintain weight within 5% of baseline B. Pt's electrolyte balance will be WNL	III. A. Assess baseline nutritional status, including electrolytes B. Assess bowel elimination status and monitor nutritional and elimination status closely postoperatively C. Discuss management strategies with MD
IV. A. Changes in BP will be detected early	IV. A. Assess baseline vital signs and monitor closely during postoperative phase B. Discuss any abnormalities with MD
V. A. Pt will be comfortable	V. A. Assess baseline comfort level, and monitor closely during postoperative course B. Provide physical and mental comfort measures C. If ineffective, discuss alternative strategies with MD for symptom management

Tamoxifen citrate
(Nolvadex)

> *Class:* Antiestrogen

MECHANISM OF ACTION

Nonsteroidal antiestrogen that binds to estrogen receptors, forming an abnormal complex that migrates to the cell nucleus and inhibits DNA synthesis.

METABOLISM

Well absorbed from gastrointestinal tract and metabolized by liver. Undergoes enterohepatic circulation, prolonging blood levels. Excreted in feces. Elimination half-life is 7 days.

DOSAGE/RANGE

20–80 mg orally daily (most often, 20-mg BID)

DRUG PREPARATION

Available in 10-mg tablets

DRUG ADMINISTRATION

Oral

SPECIAL CONSIDERATIONS

Measurement of estrogen receptors in tumor may be important in predicting tumor response and should be performed at same time as biopsy and before antiestrogen treatment is started.

Avoid antacids within 2 hours of taking entericcoated tablets.

A "flare" reaction with bony pain and hypercalcemia may occur. Such reactions are short-lived and usually result in a tumor response if therapy is continued.

Tamoxifen citrate

Nursing Diagnosis	Defining Characteristics
I. *Potential for sexual dysfunction*	I. A. May cause menstural irregularity, hot flashes, milk production in breasts, vaginal discharge and bleeding B. Symptoms occur in about 10% of pts and are usually not severe enough to discontinue therapy
II. *Potential for alteration in comfort*	II. A. May cause "flare" reaction initially (bone and tumor pain, transient increase in tumor size) B. Nausea and vomiting and anorexia may occur
III. *Potential for sensory/ perceptual alteration*	III. A. Retinopathy has been reported with high doses B. Corneal changes (infrequent), decreased visual acuity, and blurred vision have occurred C. Headache, dizziness, and light-headedness are rare
IV. *Potential for infection and bleeding related to bone marrow depression*	IV. A. Mild transient leukopenia and thrombocytopenia occur rarely
V. *Potential for skin integrity impairment*	V. A. Skin rash, alopecia, and peripheral edema are rare
VI. *Potential for injury related to hypercalcemia*	VI. A. Hypercalcemia uncommon

Expected Outcomes	**Nursing Interventions**
I. A. Pt and significant other will identify strategies for coping with sexual dysfunction	I. A. As appropriate, explore with pt and significant other issues of reproductive and sexuality pattern and impact drug may have B. Discuss strategies to preserve sexual and reproductive health
II. A. Pt will identify s/s of flare reaction and strategies to cope with it B. Pt will avoid nausea and vomiting and anorexia C. Nausea and vomiting and anorexia, should they occur, will be minimal	II. A. Inform pt of possibility of flare reactions and s/s to be aware of; encourage pt to report any s/s B. Inform pt of possibility of nausea and vomiting and anorexia C. Encourage small, frequent feedings of high-calorie, high-protein foods
III. A. Visual disturbance and CNS symptoms will be identified early	III. A. Obtain visual assessment prior to starting therapy B. Encourage pt to report any visual changes C. Instruct pt to report headache, dizziness, light-headedness
IV. A. Pt will be without s/s of infection or bleeding	IV. A. Monitor CBC, platelet count prior to therapy and after therapy has begun B. Instruct pt in self-assessment of s/s of infection or bleeding
V. A. Skin integrity will be maintained	V. A. Assess pt for s/s of hair loss, edema, and skin rash B. Instruct pt to report any of these symptoms C. Discuss with pt the impact of skin changes
VI. A. Serum calcium will remain within normal limits	VI. A. Obtain serum calcium levels prior to therapy and at regular intervals during therapy B. Instruct pt in s/s of hypercalcemia: nausea, vomiting, weakness, constipation, loss of muscle tone, malaise, decreased urine output

Teniposide
(Vumon, VM-26)

Class: Plant alkaloid, a derivative of the mandrake plant
(*Mandragora officinarum*); investigational

MECHANISM OF ACTION

Cell cycle-specific in late S phase, early G_2 phase, causing arrest of cell
division in mitosis. Inhibits uptake of thymidine into DNA, so
DNA synthesis is impaired.

METABOLISM

Drug binds extensively to serum protein. Metabolized by the liver and
excreted in bile and urine.

DOSAGE/RANGE

100 mg/m^2 weekly for 6–8 weeks
50 mg/m^2 twice a week × 4

DRUG PREPARATION

Available investigationally in 10-mg/ml 5-ml ampules. Add desired
NS for injection, or 5% dextrose in water, to reach final concentration of 0.1–0.4 mg/ml (stable for 24 hours) or 1 mg/ml (stable
for 4 hours).

DRUG ADMINISTRATION

Do not administer the solution if a precipitate is noted.

Use only non-DEHP containers such as glass or polyolefin plastic bags or containers.

Do not use polyvinyl chloride IV bags, as the DEHP will leach into the solution.

Administer over at least 30–60 minutes.

SPECIAL CONSIDERATIONS

Rapid infusion, less than 30 minutes, may cause hypotension and sudden death.

Chemical phlebitis may occur if drug is not properly diluted or if it is infused too rapidly.

Severe myelosuppression may occur.

Hypersensitivity reactions, including anaphylaxis-like symptoms, may occur with initial or repeated doses.

Drug is prepared by the manufacturer with polyoxyethylated castor oil and dehydrated alcohol, which may stimulate hypersensitivity.

Reduce doses of tolbutamide, sodium salicylate, or sulfamethizole if given concurrently.

Heparin causes precipitate.

Teniposide

Nursing Diagnosis	Defining Characteristics
I. *Potential for injury during drug administration related to* A. Hypotension	I. A. Hypotension may occur during rapid infusion
B. Anaphylaxis	B. 1. Rarely occurs; may be characterized by fever, dyspnea, lumbar pain, progressive hypotension 2. May respond to drug discontinuance and IV hydrocortisone

Expected Outcomes	Nursing Interventions
I. A. Hypotension will be prevented	I. A. 1. Monitor BP prior to drug administration and periodically during infusion at least during first drug administration 2. Infuse over at least 30–60 mins

B. Anaphylaxis, if it occurs, will be managed successfully	B. 1. Have anaphylaxis tray with corticosteroids, antihistamines, epinephrine nearby when chemotherapy is administered
	2. Monitor pt closely during infusion
	3. Review standing orders for management of allergic reactions (hypersensitivity and anaphylaxis) as per institutional policy and procedure
	4. Prior to drug administration, obtain baseline vital signs and record mental status
	5. Observe for following s/s, usually occurring within the first 15 mins of infusion:
	a. *Subjective*
	   (1) generalized itching
	   (2) nausea
	   (3) chest tightness
	   (4) crampy abdominal pain
	   (5) agitation
	   (6) anxiety
	   (7) sense of impending doom
	   (8) wheeziness
	   (9) desire to urinate or defecate
	   (10) dizziness
	   (11) chills
	b. *Objective*
	   (1) flushed appearance (angioedema of the face, neck, eyelids, hands, feet)

Teniposide *Continued*

Nursing Diagnosis	Defining Characteristics
B. Anaphylaxis	
II. *Potential for infection and bleeding related to bone marrow depression*	II. A. Dose-limiting toxicity B. Leukopenia; thrombocytopenia may also occur C. Nadir 3–14 days (~7 days) D. Dose reduction indicated for pts heavily pretreated with radiation or chemotherapy
III. *Altered nutrition, less than body requirements related to* A. Nausea and vomiting	III. A. May occur, but are usually mild

Expected Outcomes	**Nursing Interventions**

	(2) localized or generalized urticaria
	     (3) respiratory distress ± wheezing
	     (4) hypotension
	     (5) cyanosis
	  6. For generalized allergic response, stop infusion and notify MD
	  7. Place pt in supine position to promote perfusion of visceral organs
	  8. Monitor vital signs
	  9. Provide emotional reassurance to pt and family
	 10. Maintain patient airway and have equipment ready for CPR if needed
	 11. Document incident
	 12. Discuss with MD desensitization versus drug discontinuance for further dose

II. A. Pt will be without s/s of infection or bleeding
     B. Early s/s of infection or bleeding will be identified
	II. A. Monitor platelet count prior to drug administration, assess for s/s of infection or bleeding; assess nadir counts
	     B. Instruct pt in self-assessment techniques for infection or bleeding
	     C. Dose reduction may be necessary based on nadir counts, history of previous XRT/chemotherapy, altered hepatic function
	     D. Transfuse with red cells, platelets per MD order

III. A. Pt will be without nausea and vomiting	III. A. 1. Premedicate with antiemetic and continue prophylactically ×24 hrs to prevent nausea and vomiting, at least for first treatment

Teniposide *Continued*

Nursing Diagnosis	Defining Characteristics
B. Hepatic dysfunction	B. Mild elevation of liver function tests may occur
IV. *Potential for impaired skin integrity related to* A. Alopecia	IV. A. Occurs uncommonly (9–30%) and is reversible
B. Irritation	B. Phlebitis or perivascular irritation may occur if drug is too concentrated or is infused too rapidly
V. *Potential for alteration in cardiac output*	V. A. Rarely, palpitations may occur
VI. *Potential for sensory/ perceptual alterations related to neurological toxicity*	VI. A. Peripheral neuropathies may occur and are mild

Expected Outcomes	**Nursing Interventions**
	2. Encourage small, frequent feedings of cool, bland foods and liquids
B. Hepatic dysfunction will be identified early	B. 1. Monitor SGOT, SGPT, LDH, alkaline phosphatase, and bilirubin prior to drug administration
	2. Notify MD of any elevations
IV. A. 1. Pt will verbalize feelings re hair loss	IV. A. 1. Discuss with pt impact of hair loss
2. Pt will identify strategies to cope with changes in body image	2. Suggest wig as appropriate prior to actual hair loss
	3. Explore with pt response to actual hair loss and plan strategies to minimize distress (e.g., wig, scarf, cap)
B. Phlebitis, irritation will be minimal	B. Use careful venipuncture technique and administer drug over 30–60 mins, diluted to at least 5 volumes as per manufacturer's specifications
V. A. Early cardiac rhythm abnormalities will be identified	V. A. Monitor heart rate, noting rhythm, when administering drug
	B. Notify MD of any irregularity
	C. EKG to identify irregular rhythm
VI. A. Peripheral neuropathy will be identified early	VI. A. Assess motor and sensory function prior to therapy
B. Pt will verbalize feelings re discomfort and dysfunction related to neuropathy and identify alternative coping strategies	B. Encourage pt to verbalize feelings re discomfort and sensory loss if these occur
	C. Assist pt to discuss alternative coping strategies

6-Thioguanine
(Thioguanine, Tabloid, 6-TG)

Class: Thiopurine antimetabolite

MECHANISM OF ACTION

Converts to monophosphate nucleotides and inhibits de novo purine synthesis. The nucleotides are also incorporated into DNA. Cell cycle phase-specific (S phase).

Thioguanine interferes with nucleic acid bio-synthesis, resulting in sequential blockage of the synthesis and utilization of the purine nucleotides.

METABOLISM

Absorption is incomplete and variable orally. Is metabolized in the liver by deamination and methylation. Metabolites are excreted in the urine and feces. Plasma half-life is 80–90 minutes.

DOSAGE/RANGE

Children and adults: 100 mg/m^2 orally every 12 hours for 5–10 days, usually in combination with cytarabine

100 mg/m^2 IV daily $\times$ 5 days

1–3 mg/kg orally daily

DRUG PREPARATION

Available in 40-mg tablets.
Reconstitute 100-mg vial in 15 ml NS.

DRUG ADMINISTRATION

IV bolus

SPECIAL CONSIDERATIONS

Oral dose to be given on empty stomach to facilitate complete absorption.
Dose is titrated to avoid excessive stomatitis and diarrhea.
6-Thioguanine can be used in full doses with allopurinol.

6-Thioguanine

Nursing Diagnosis	Defining Characteristics
I. *Altered nutrition, less than body requirements related to*	I.
A. Nausea and vomiting	A. Nausea and vomiting occur uncommonly, especially in children, but are dose related
B. Anorexia	B. Rare
C. Stomatitis	C. Rare, but most common with high doses
D. Hepatotoxicity	D. Rare, but may be associated with hepatic venoocclusive disease or jaundice

II. *Potential for infection and bleeding related to bone marrow depression*	II. A. Bone marrow depression occurs 1–4 weeks after treatment
	   B. Leukopenia and thrombocytopenia are most common
	   C. Drug may have prolonged or delayed nadir

III. *Potential for sensory/perceptual alterations*	III. A. Loss of vibratory sensation, unsteady gait may occur

Expected Outcomes	Nursing Interventions
I. A. 1. Pt will be without nausea and vomiting 2. Nausea and vomiting, should they occur, will be minimal	I. A. 1. Treat symptomatically with antiemetics 2. Encourage small, frequent feedings of cool, bland foods and liquids 3. If vomiting occurs, assess for fluid and electrolyte imbalance; monitor I&O and daily weights if pt is hospitalized
B. Pt will maintain baseline weight ± 5%	B. 1. Encourage small, frequent feedings of favorite foods, especially high-calorie, high-protein foods 2. Encourage use of spices 3. Weekly weights
C. Oral mucous membranes will remain intact and without infection	C. 1. Teach oral assessment and oral hygiene regimen 2. Encourage pt to report early stomatitis 3. Provide pain relief measures if indicated
D. Hepatotoxicity will be identified early	D. 1. Monitor LFT's prior to drug dose 2. Assess pt prior to and during treatment for s/s of hepatotoxicity
II. A. Pt will be without s/s of infection or bleeding B. Early s/s of infection or bleeding will be identified	II. A. Monitor CBC, platelet count prior to drug administration, as well as s/s of infection or bleeding B. Instruct pt in self-assessment of s/s of infection or bleeding C. Administer platelet, red cell transfusions per MD order
III. A. Neurological toxicity will be identified early	III. A. Assess vibratory sensation, gait before each dose and between treatments B. Report changes to MD C. Encourage pt to report any changes

Thiotepa
(Triethylene Thiophosphoramide)

Class: Alkylating agent

MECHANISM OF ACTION

Selectively reacts with DNA phosphate groups to produce chromo-some cross-linkage with blocking of nucleoprotein synthesis. Acts as a polyfunctional alkylating agent. Cell cycle phase-nonspecific. Mimics radiation-induced injury.

METABOLISM

Rapidly cleared following IV administration; 60% of dose is elimi-nated in urine within 24–72 hours. Slow onset of action, slowly bound to tissues, extensively metabolized.

DOSAGE/RANGE

Intravenous
8 mg/m^2 (0.2 mg/kg) IV every day × 5 days, repeated every 3–4 weeks
30–60 mg IV, IM, or SQ once a week, depending on WBC
Intracavitary
Bladder: 60 mg in 60 ml sterile water once a week for 3–4 weeks

DRUG PREPARATION

Add sterile water to vial of lyophilized powder.

Further dilute with NS or D_5W.

Do not use solution unless it is clear.

Refrigerate vial until use (reconstituted solution is stable for 5 days).

DRUG ADMINISTRATION

IV, IM; intracavitary; intra-tumor; intra-arterial

SPECIAL CONSIDERATIONS

Hypersensitivity reactions have occurred with this drug.

Is an irritant; should be given via a sidearm of a running IV.

Increased neuromuscular blockage when given with nondepolarizing
   muscle relaxants.

Thiotepa

Nursing Diagnosis	Defining Characteristics
I. *Potential for infection and bleeding related to bone marrow depression*	I. A. Nadir is 5–30 days after drug administration B. Thrombocytopenia and leukopenia may occur C. Anemia may occur with prolonged use D. May be cumulative toxicity, with recovery of bone marrow in 40–50 days E. Thrombocytopenia is dose limiting
II. *Altered nutrition, less than body requirements related to* A. Nausea and vomiting B. Anorexia	II. A. 1. Nausea and vomiting occur in 10–15% of pts 2. Dose dependent 3. Occur 6–12 hrs after drug dose B. Occurs occasionally
III. *Sexual dysfunction*	III. A. Drug is mutagenic B. Sterility may be reversible and incomplete C. Amenorrhea often reverses in 6–8 months

Expected Outcomes	Nursing Interventions
I. A. Pt will be without s/s of infection or bleeding B. Early s/s of infection or bleeding will be detected	I. A. Monitor CBC, platelet count prior to drug administration; monitor for s/s of infection or bleeding B. Instruct pt in self-assessment of s/s of infection or bleeding C. Administer red cell and platelet transfusions per MD order
II. A. 1. Pt will be without nausea and vomiting 2. Nausea and vomiting, if they occur, will be minimal B. Pt will maintain baseline weight ±5%	II. A. 1. Premedicate with antiemetics, especially with parenteral high dose; continue antiemetics at least 12 hrs after drug is given 2. Encourage small, frequent feedings of cool, bland, dry foods B. 1. Encourage small, frequent feedings of favorite foods, especially high-calorie, high-protein foods 2. Encourage use of spices 3. Weekly weights
III. A. Pt and significant other will identify coping strategies to deal with sexual dysfunction	III. A. As appropriate, explore with pt and significant other issues of reproductive and sexuality pattern and anticipated impact chemotherapy will have B. Discuss strategies to preserve sexuality and reproductive health (e.g., sperm banking)

Thiotepa *Continued*

Nursing Diagnosis	Defining Characteristics
IV. *Potential for injury related to*	
A. Allergic reaction	IV. A. Allergic responses may occur rarely: hives, bronchospasm, skin rash (dermatitis)
B. Secondary malignancies	B. Secondary malignancies may occur with prolonged therapy
V. *Alteration in comfort*	V. A. Dizziness, headache, fever, and local pain may occur

Expected Outcomes	Nursing Interventions
IV. A. Allergic responses will be detected early and treated	IV. A. 1. Assess for s/s of allergic response during drug administration 2. Stop drug if bronchospasm occurs and notify MD 3. Discuss symptomatic treatment with MD
B. Secondary malignancy, if it occurs, will be detected early	B. Instruct pt receiving prolonged therapy in importance of regular health maintenance examinations during and after therapy by primary care provider and oncologist
V. A. Distress will be minimal	V. A. Assess for alterations in comfort B. Treat symptomatically

Topotecan hydrochloride for injection
(Hycamptin)

Class: Topoisomerase inhibitor

MECHANISM OF ACTION

Causes single-strand breaks in DNA to permit relaxation of the DNA
helix before DNA replication. Topotecan binds to the topoisomerase I DNA complex, thus preventing repair of the breaks, and
ultimately DNA synthesis, and leads to cell death.

METABOLISM

Thirty percent of the drug is excreted in the urine. Moderate renal impairment leads to a 34% decrease in plasma clearance of the drug
so a dose reduction is necessary. Minor metabolism occurs in the
liver.

DOSAGE/RANGE

1.5 mg/m^2 IV qd × 5, repeated q 21 days

DRUG PREPARATION

Reconstitute 4-mg-vial with 4 ml sterile water for injection. Further
dilute in 0.9% sodium chloride or 5% dextrose, and use immediately.

DRUG ADMINISTRATION

Infuse over 30 minutes. Baseline ANC for initial course must be $\geq 1500/mm^3$ and platelet count $\geq 100,000/mm^3$, and for subsequent courses, ANC $\geq 1000/mm^3$, platelets $\geq 100,000/mm^3$, and hemoglobin ≥ 9 mg/dl.

LAB EFFECTS/INTERFERENCE

Decrease in CBC; increase in LFTs, RFTs

DRUG INTERACTIONS

None known

SPECIAL CONSIDERATIONS

G-CSF (Neupogen) may be required in neutro-penia develops first cycle.

Dose modifications recommended by manufacturer:

Renal impairment: mild = creatinine clearance (cr cl) 40–60 ml/min, dose is 0.75 mg/m^2; moderate = cr cl 29–39 ml/min, consider drug discontinuance.

Hematologic toxicity: severe neutropenia, dose reduce by 0.25 mg/m^2 for subsequent doses or use G-CSF beginning on day 6 (24 hours after last dose of drug).

Minimum of 4 courses needed, as clinical responses occur 9–12 weeks after beginning of therapy.

Indicated for the treatment of relapsed or refractory metastatic ovarian cancer, but has activity in many solid tumors.

Topotecan hydrochloride for injection

Nursing Diagnosis	Defining Characteristics
I. *Infection and bleeding related to bone marrow depression*	I. A. Dose limiting toxicity B. Grade 4 neutropenia seen during first course in 60% of pts. Febrile neutropenia or sepsis may occur in 26% of pts C. Nadir occurs on day 11 D. Grade 4 thrombocytopenia occurs in 26% of pts (platelet count < 25,000/mm^3) E. Platelet nadir occurs on day 15
II. *Potential for activity intolerance related to anemia-induced fatigue*	II. A. Severe anemia (Hgb < 8 gm/dl) occurs in 40% of pts B. 56% of pts require transfusions

Expected Outcomes	Nursing Interventions
I. A. Pt will be without s/s of infection or bleeding	I. A. Monitor CBC, platelet count prior to drug administration, as well as start of infection and bleeding. Assess baseline renal function prior to each cycle B. Teach s/s of infection and bleeding, pt self-assessment, and to call or come to ER if T > 100.5 or per institutional policy, and s/s of bleeding. Teach pt to avoid aspirin or aspirin containing OTC medicines, NSAIDs, and other medicines without talking to RN or MD first C. Teach pt/family retionale for G-CSF, and how to prepare and administer medicine if ordered to prevent febrile neutropenia
II. A. Pt will be able to do desired activities B. Early fatigue related to anemia will resolve	II. A. Monitor hemoglobin, hematocrit B. Teach pt/family rationale for EPO, and how to prepare and administer injection if ordered C. Transfuse per MD for hematocrit < 25, s/s of severe anemia D. Teach pt diet high in iron, folic acid; teach self-administration of folic acid, iron medications as ordered E. Teach pt to alternate rest and activity periods

Topotecan hydrochloride for injection *Continued*

Nursing Diagnosis	Defining Characteristics
III. *Alteration in nutrition, less than body requirements related to*	
A. Nausea and vomiting	III. A. 1. Nausea occurs in 77% of pts and vomiting in 58% of pts without premedication 2. Abdominal pain occurs in 33% of pts
B. Diarrhea	B. Diarrhea occurs in 39% of pts
C. Elevated LFTs	C. Elevated LFTs occur in 5% of pts (AST [SGOT], ALT [SGPT])
IV. *Potential for hepatotoxicity related preexisting hepatic insufficiency*	IV. A. There may be increased drug toxicity in pts with low serum protein and hepatic dysfunction

Expected Outcomes	Nursing Interventions

III. A. 1. Pt will be without nausea and vomiting
        2. Nausea and vomiting, should they occur, will be minimal
	III. A. 1. Premedicate with antiemetics, such as a serotonin-antagonist to prevent nausea and vomiting
	        2. Encourage small, frequent feedings of cool, bland foods and liquids
	        3. Assess for symptoms of fluid and electrolyte imbalance; monitor daily weights for 5-day course

B. Pt will have minimal diarrhea	B. 1. Assess pt's bowel elimination pattern; guaiac all stools
	     2. Encourage pt to report onset of diarrhea
	     3. Administer or teach pt to self-administer antidiarrheal medications

C. Changes in LFTs will be identified early	C. 1. Assess baseline LFTs and monitor periodically during therapy 2. Discuss any elevations with physician
IV. A. Evidence of hepatotoxicity will be identified early	IV. A. Assess baseline serum albumin, LFTs prior to first dose, and during treatment B. If hepatotoxicity develops, assess for increased drug toxicity and discuss dose reduction with physician

Vinblastine
(Velban)

Class: Plant alkaloid extracted from the periwinkle plant (*Vinca rosea*)

MECHANISM OF ACTION

Drug binds to microtubular proteins, thus arresting mitosis during metaphase; may inhibit RNA, DNA, and protein synthesis. Active in S and M phases (cell cycle phase-specific).

METABOLISM

About 10% of drug is excreted in feces. Vinblastine is partially metabolized by the liver. Minimal amount of the drug is excreted in urine and bile. Dose modification may be necessary in the presence of hepatic failure.

DOSAGE/RANGE

0.1 mg/kg or 6 mg/m^2 IV weekly: continuous infusion 1.4–1.8 mg/day × 5 days

DRUG PREPARATION

Available in 10-mg vials. Store in refrigerator until use.

DRUG ADMINISTRATION

IV push or by continuous infusion. When given as a continuous infusion, must be given via central line, as drug is a potent vesicant.

SPECIAL CONSIDERATIONS

Drug is a vesicant. Give through a running IV to avoid extravasation.

Dose modification may be necessary in the presence of hepatic failure.

Decreased pharmacologic effects of phenytoin when given with this drug.

Increases cellular uptake of methotrexate by certain malignant cells when administered sequentially, but less so than vincristine.

Vinblastine

Nursing Diagnosis	Defining Characteristics
I. *Potential for infection and bleeding related to bone marrow depression*	I. A. May cause severe BMD B. Nadir 4–10 days C. Neutrophils greatly affected D. In pts with prior XRT or chemotherapy, thrombocytopenia may be severe
II. *Potential for sensory/ perceptual alterations*	II. A. Occur less frequently than with vincristine B. Occur in pts receiving prolonged or high-dose therapy C. Symptoms: paresthesias, peripheral neuropathy, depression, headache, malaise, jaw pain, urinary retention, tachycardia, orthostatic hypotension, seizures D. Rare ocular changes: diplopia, ptosis, photophobia, oculomotor dysfunction, optic neuropathy
III. *Potential for constipation*	III. A. Constipation results from neurotoxicity (central) and is less common than with vincristine B. Risk factors: high dose (> 20 mg) C. May lead to adynamic ileus, abdominal pain
IV. *Altered nutrition, less than body requirements related to* A. Nausea and vomiting	IV. A. Rarely occur

Expected Outcomes	**Nursing Interventions**
I. A. Pt will be without s/s of infection or bleeding B. Early s/s of infection or bleeding will be identified	I. A. Monitor CBC, platelet count prior to drug administration B. Assess for s/s of infection or bleeding C. Instruct pt in self-assessment of s/s of infection or bleeding D. Dose reduction if hepatic dysfunction: 50% if bilirubin > 1.5 mg/dl; 75% if bilirubin > 3.0 mg/dl E. Administer red cell, platelet transfusions as ordered
II. A. Sensory/perceptual changes will be identified early B. Dysfunction will be minimized C. Discomfort will be minimized	II. A. Assess sensory/perceptual changes prior to each drug dose, especially if dose is high (> 10 mg) or pt is receiving prolonged therapy B. Notify MD of alterations C. Discuss with pt impact changes have had and strategies to minimize dysfunction and decrease distress
III. A. Constipation will be prevented B. Early s/s of adynamic ileus will be identified	III. A. Assess bowel elimination pattern after each drug dose, especially if dose > 20 mg B. Teach pt to promote bowel evacuation by fluids (3 l/day), high-fiber, bulky foods, exercise, stool softeners C. Suggest laxative if unable to move bowels at least once a day D. Instruct pt to report abdominal pain
IV. A. 1. Pt will be without nausea and vomiting 2. Nausea and vomiting, if they occur, will be minimal	IV. A. 1. Premedicate with antiemetics and continue prophylactically × 24 hrs to prevent nausea and vomiting, at least for the first treatment 2. Encourage small, frequent feedings of cool, bland foods and liquids

Vinblastine *Continued*

Nursing Diagnosis	Defining Characteristics
B. Stomatitis	B. Occurs occasionally; may be severe
C. Diarrhea	C. Occasional, infrequent, and mild
V. *Potential for impaired skin integrity related to* A. Alopecia	V. A. 1. Reversible and mild 2. Occurs in 45–50% of pts receiving drug
B. Extravasation	B. Drug is a potent vesicant and can cause irritation and necrosis if infiltrated

Expected Outcomes	Nursing Interventions
	3. Assess for symptoms of fluid and electrolyte imbalance; monitor I&O, daily weights if inpatient
B. Oral mucous membranes will remain intact and without infection	B. 1. Teach pt oral assessment 2. Teach, reinforce teaching, re oral hygiene regimens 3. Encourage pt to report early stomatitis 4. Provide pain relief measures if indicated (e.g., topical anesthetics)
C. Pt will have minimal diarrhea	C. 1. Encourage pt to report onset of diarrhea 2. Administer or teach pt to self-administer antidiarrheal medication 3. Suggest diet modification
V. A. 1. Pt will verbalize feelings re hair loss 2. Pt will identify strategies to cope with changes in body image	V. A. 1. Discuss with pt impact of hair loss 2. Suggest wig as appropriate prior to actual hair loss 3. Explore with pt response to actual hair loss and plan strategies to minimize distress (i.e., wig, scarf, cap)
B. 1. Extravasation will be avoided 2. Skin will heal completely if extravasation occurs	B. 1. For safe administration of vesicant 2. Use careful technique during venipuncture 3. Administer vesicant through freely flowing IV, constantly monitoring IV site and pt response 4. Nurse should be *thoroughly* familiar with institutional policy and procedure for administration of a vesicant agent

Vinblastine *Continued*

Nursing Diagnosis	Defining Characteristics
B. Extravasation	
C. Rash	C. Uncommon

Expected Outcomes	Nursing Interventions
	5. If vesicant drug is administered as a continuous infusion, drug must be given through a patient central line
	6. If extravasation is suspected: a. Stop drug administered b. Aspirate any residual drug and blood from IV tubing, IV catheter/needle, and IV site if possible c. If drug infiltration is suspected, manufacturer suggests the following after withdrawing any remaining drug from IV: local installation of hyaluronidase, apply moderate heat
	7. Assess site regularly for pain, progression of erythema, induration, and evidence of necrosis
	8. When in doubt about whether drug is infiltrating, *treat as an infiltration*
	9. Teach pt to assess site and notify MD if condition worsens
	10. Arrange next clinic visit for assessment of site depending on drug, amount infiltrated, extent of potential injury, and pt variables
	11. Document in pt's record as per institutional policy and procedure
C. Pt will identify strategies to cope with rash	C. Assess impact of rash on pt (body image, comfort) and treat symptomatically

Vinblastine *Continued*

Nursing Diagnosis	Defining Characteristics
VI. *Potential for sexual dysfunction*	VI. A. Drug is possibly teratogenic B. Likely to cause azoospermia in men

Expected Outcomes	Nursing Interventions
VI. A. Pt and significant other will identify strategies to cope with sexual dysfunction	VI. A. As appropriate, explore with pt and significant other issues of reproductive and sexuality pattern and anticipated impact chemotherapy will have B. Discuss strategies to preserve reproductive health (e.g., sperm banking)

Vincristine
(Oncovin)

Class: Plant alkaloid extracted from the periwinkle plant (*Vinca rosea*)

MECHANISM OF ACTION

Drug binds to microtubular proteins, thus arresting mitosis during metaphase. Cell cycle phase-specific in M and S phases.

METABOLISM

The primary route for excretion is via the liver, with about 70% of the drug being excreted in feces and bile. These metabolites are a result of hepatic metabolism and biliary excretion. A small amount is excreted in the urine. Dose modification may be necessary in the presence of hepatic failure.

DOSAGE/RANGE

0.4–1.4 mg/m^2 weekly (initially limited to 2 mg per dose)

DRUG PREPARATION

Supplied in 1-mg, 2-mg, and 5-mg vials. Refrigerate vials until use.

DRUG ADMINISTRATION

IV push or as a continuous infusion over 24 hours. When given as a
   continuous infusion, should be administered through a central
   line, as drug is a potent vesicant.

SPECIAL CONSIDERATIONS

Drug is a vesicant. Give through a running IV to avoid extravasation.

Dose modification may be necessary in the presence of hepatic failure.

Decreased bioavailability of digoxin when given with this drug.

Increased cellular uptake of methotrexate by some malignant cells
   when given sequentially.

Vincristine

Nursing Diagnosis	Defining Characteristics
I. *Potential for sensory/ perceptual alterations related to*	
A. Peripheral neuropathies	I. A. 1. Peripheral neuropathies occur as a result of toxicity to nerve fibers 2. Absent deep tension reflexes 3. Numbness, weakness, myalgias, cramping 4. Late severe motor difficulties 5. Reversal or discontinuance of therapy necessary 6. Increased risk in elderly
B. Cranial nerve damage and other nerve involvement	B. 1. Cranial nerve dysfunction may occur (rare) 2. Jaw pain (trigeminal neuralgia) 3. Diplopia 4. Vocal cord paresis 5. Mental depression 6. Metallic taste
C. Constipation	C. 1. Autonomic neuropathy may lead to constipation and paralytic ileus 2. A concurrent use of vinblastine, narcotic analgesics, or cholinergic medication may increase risk of constipation

Expected Outcomes	**Nursing Interventions**
I. A. 1. Sensory and perceptual changes will be identified early 2. Dysfunction will be minimized 3. Discomfort will be minimized	I. A. 1. Assess sensory and perceptual changes prior to each drug dose (i.e., presence of numbness or tingling of fingertips or toes) 2. Assess for loss of deep tendon reflexes: foot drop, slapping gait 3. Assess for motor difficulties: clumsiness of hands, difficulty climbing stairs (buttoning shirt, walking on heels) 4. Notify MD of alterations: discuss holding drug if loss of deep tendon reflexes occurs 5. Discuss with pt impact alterations have had and strategies to minimize dysfunction and decrease distress 6. Discuss with pt type of alteration: memory, sensory/perceptual, temporary and reversible when drug stopped
B. Symptoms of nerve dysfunction will be identified early	B. 1. Assess pt for s/s of nerve dysfunction before each dose 2. Notify MD of any changes
C. 1. Constipation will be prevented 2. Early s/s of paralytic ileus will be identified	I. C. 1. Assess bowel elimination pattern prior to each chemotherapy administration 2. Teach pt to include bulky and high-fiber foods in diet, increase fluids to 3 L/day, and exercise moderately to promote elimination 3. Suggest stool softeners if needed

Vincristine *Continued*

Nursing Diagnosis	Defining Characteristics
C. Constipation	
II. *Potential for impaired skin integrity related to* A. Alopecia and subsequent body image disturbance	II. A. 1. Complete hair loss occurs in 12–45% of pts 2. Both men and women are at risk for body image disturbance 3. Hair will grow back
B. Dermatitis	B. Uncommon
C. Extravasation	C. Drug is potent vesicant, causing irritation and necrosis if infiltrated

Expected Outcomes	**Nursing Interventions**
	4. Teach pt to use laxative if unable to move bowels at least once every 2 days 5. Instruct pt to report abdominal pain
II. A. Pt will verbalize feelings about hair loss and identify strategies to cope with change in body image	II. A. 1. Discuss with pt anticipated impact of hair loss; suggest wig or toupee as appropriate prior to actual hair loss 2. Explore with pt response to hair loss, if it occurs, and strategies to minimize distress (i.e., wig, scarf, cap)
B. Pt will identify coping strategies	B. 1. Assess impact on pt: body image, comfort 2. Discuss strategies to minimize distress

C. 1. Extravasation will be avoided
2. Skin will heal completely if drug is extravasated
	C. 1. Use careful technique during venipuncture
	2. Administer vesicant through freely flowing IV, constantly monitoring IV site and pt response
	3. Nurse should be *thoroughly* familiar with institutional policy and procedure for administration of a vesicant agent
	4. If vesicant drug is administered as a continuous infusion, drug must be given through a patent central line
	5. If extravasation is suspected:
	  a. Stop drug being administered
	  b. Aspirate any residual drug and blood from IV tubing, IV catheter/needle and IV site if possible

Vincristine *Continued*

Nursing Diagnosis	Defining Characteristics
C. Extravasation	
III. *Potential for infection and bleeding related to bone marrow depression*	III. A. Rare myelosuppression; mild when it occurs B. May have cumulative bone marrow depression over time, requiring transfusion C. Nadir 10–14 days after treatment begins
IV. *Potential for sexual dysfunction*	IV. A. Impotence may occur related to neurotoxicity

Expected Outcomes	**Nursing Interventions**
	c. If drug infiltration is suspected, manufacturer suggests the following after withdrawing any remaining drug from tubing: local injection of hyaluronidase, apply moderate heat
	6. Assess site regularly for pain, progression of erythema, induration, and evidence of necrosis
	7. When in doubt about whether drug is infiltrating, *treat as an infiltration*
	8. Teach pt to assess site and notify MD if condition worsens
	9. Arrange next clinic visit for assessment of site depending on drug, amount infiltrated, extent of potential injury, and pt variables
	10. Document in pt's record as per institutional policy and procedure
III. A. Pt will be without bleeding or infection B. Early s/s of bleeding or infection will be detected	III. A. Monitor WBC, hematocrit, platelets prior to drug administration B. Dose reduction if hepatic dysfunction: 50% reduction if bilirubin >1.5 mg/dl; 75% reduction if bilirubin >3.0mg/dl
IV. A. Pt and significant other will identify strategies to cope with sexual dysfunction	IV. A. As appropriate, explore with pt and significant other issues of reproductive and sexuality pattern and impact chemotherapy may have B. Discuss strategies to preserve sexual health (i.e., alternative expressions of sexuality) C. Reassure pt that impotency, if it occurs, is usually temporary and reversible after drug discontinuance

Vinorelbine
(Navelbine)

Class: Semisynthetic vinca alkaloid derived from vinblastine

MECHANISM OF ACTION

Inhibits mitosis at metaphase by interfering with microtubule assembly. Also appears to interfere with some aspects of cellular metabolism, including cellular respiration and nucleic acid biosynthesis. Cell cycle–specific.

METABOLISM

Slow elimination; extensive tissue binding (80% bound to plasma proteins); metabolized by the liver. Terminal half-life is 27–43 hours. Excreted in feces (46%) and urine (18%).

DOSAGE/RANGE

30 mg/m^2 IV weekly or in combination with 120 mg/m^2 cisplatin given on days 1 and 29, then every 6 weeks. Investigationally, 80 mg/m^2 po weekly.

DRUG PREPARATION

Available as 10-mg/ml solution in 1-ml or 5-ml vials. Further dilute in 75–250 ml 0.9% sodium chloride or 5% dextrose in water. Final concentration should be 1.5–3 mg/ml for syringe and 0.5–2 mg/ml for IV bolus administration. Stable for 24 hours at room temperature. Oral preparation available as 40-mg gelatin capsules.

DRUG ADMINISTRATION

Drug is a vesicant. It is administered IV over 6–10 minutes by slow IV push via syringe into the sidearm closest to the IV bag of a freely flowing IV, followed by a 75–125 ml flush or by IV bolus infusion via a central line. Refer to individual hospital policy and procedure for vesicant administration.

Oral capsule should be taken on an empty stomach at bedtime.

(Vinorelbine continued)

SPECIAL CONSIDERATIONS

There has been a 33% response rate in non-small cell lung cancer when used as single agent and a 65% response in combination with cisplatin, 5-fluorouracil, and leucovorin.

Overall response rate in metastatic breast cancer was 45%, with 20% complete responses.

Increased nausea, vomiting, and diarrhea with oral administration of capsules.

Drug is a vesicant, and as with other vinca alkaloids, hyaluronidase should be administered if extravasation is suspected.

Drug is embryotoxic and mutagenic, so female patients of childbearing age should use contraception.

Administer cautiously in patients with hepatic insufficiency.

Dose modification is necessary in the presence of hepatic dysfunction: total bilirubin 2.1–3.0 mg/dl, use 50% dose reduction (i.e., 15 mg/m^2); total bilirubin > 3.0 mg/dl, use 75% dose reduction (i.e., 7.5 mg/m^2).

Contraindicated if absolute granulocyte count (AGC) is < 1000 cells/mm^3.

Dose modification necessary for hematologic toxicity. If AGC on the day of treatment is 1000–1499 cells/m^3, use 50% dose reduction (i.e., 15 mg/m^2); drug should be held if AGC is < 1000 cells/m^3. If drug is held for 3 consecutive weeks due to AGC < 1000 cells/m^3, discontinue drug.

If patient develops granulocytopenic fever or sepsis or drug is held for granulocytopenia for 2 consecutive doses, drug dose should be reduced 25% (i.e., 22.5 mg/m^2) if AGC is > 1500 cells/mm^3; if AGC is 1000–1499 cells/mm^3, drug dose should be decreased to 11.25 mg/m^2 as per package insert.

Rarely, acute pulmonary reactions have been reported when drug is administered in combination with Mitomycin C.

Vinorelbine

Nursing Diagnosis	Defining Characteristics
I. *Infection and bleeding related to bone marrow depression*	I. A. Leukopenia is dose-limiting toxicity; bone marrow depression noncumulative and short-lived (< 7 days), with nadir 7–10 days B. Use with caution in pts with history of prior radiotherapy or chemotherapy C. Severe thrombocytopenia and anemia uncommon
II. *Potential for sensory/ perceptual alterations related to neurological toxicity*	II. A. Incidence of mild to moderate neuropathy is 25% B. Paresthesias occurs in 2–10% of pts, but incidence is increased if pt has received prior chemotherapy with vinca alkaloids or abdominal XRT C. Decreased deep tendon reflexes (6–29%) D. Constipation may occur in 29% of pts E. Reversible neuropathy
III. *Alteration in nutrition, less than body requirements related to* A. Nausea and vomiting	III. A. Incidence increases with oral dosing; mild in IV dosing, with 44% incidence; vomiting occurs in approximately 20% of pts
B. Diarrhea	B. Increased incidence with oral dosing (17%)

Expected Outcomes	**Nursing Interventions**
I. A. Pt will be without s/s of infection or bleeding B. Early s/s of infection or bleeding will be identified	I. A. Monitor CBC, platelet count prior to drug administration and postchemotherapy; assess for s/s of infection or bleeding B. Teach pt self-assessment of s/s of infection or bleeding and how to seek medical advice/care C. Dose may be held until full bone marrow recovery, then reduced 25%; see "Special Considerations" D. See "Special Considerations" for dose reduction with hepatic dysfunction E. Administer growth factor (i.e., G-CSF) > 24 hrs after drug administration, as ordered
II. A. Early s/s of neurological toxicity will be identified B. Function will be maintained	II. A. Assess baseline neuromuscular function and reassess prior to drug infusion, especially presence of paresthesias; risk is increased if drug is given concurrently with cisplatin B. Teach pt to report any changes in sensation of function C. Discuss alterations with MD D. Identify strategies to promote comfort and safety
III. A. 1. Pt will be without nausea and vomiting 2. Nausea and vomiting, if they occur, will be mild 3. Pt will maintain weight within 5% of baseline B. Pt will have minimal diarrhea	III. A. 1. Premedicate with antiemetics prior to drug administration, at least for first treatment 2. Encourage small, frequent feedings of cool, bland foods and liquids 3. Assess for symptoms of fluid/electrolyte imbalance if pt has severe nausea and vomiting 4. Monitor I&O, daily weights, lab electrolyte values B. 1. Encourage pt to report onset of diarrhea

Vinorelbine *Continued*

Nursing Diagnosis	Defining Characteristics
C. Stomatitis	C. Usually mild to moderate, with < 20% incidence
D. Hepatotoxicity	D. Transient increase in liver function studies (SGOT) occurs in 67% of pts, without clinical significance
IV. *Potential for alteration in skin integrity related to* A. Alopecia	IV. A. Incidence is 12%; reversible and mild
B. Extravasation	B. Drug is a vesicant similar to other vinca alkaloids and can cause irritation and necrosis if drug extravasates

Expected Outcomes		Nursing Interventions
		2. Administer or teach pt to self-administer antidiarrheal medication
C. Oral mucous membranes will remain intact and without infection	C.	1. Teach pt oral self-assessment
		2. Teach, reinforce teaching re oral hygiene regimen
		3. Encourage pt to report early stomatitis
		4. Provide pain relief measures if indicated (i.e., topical anesthetics)
D. Hepatic dysfunction will be identified early	D.	1. Assess liver function studies prior to drug administration and periodically during treatment
		2. Dose modification necessary for severe hepatic dysfunction (see "Special Considerations")
IV. A. Pt will verbalize feelings re hair loss and strategies to cope with change in body image	IV. A.	1. Discuss potential impact of hair loss prior to drug administration, coping strategies, and plan to minimize body image distortion (e.g., wig, scarf, cap)
		2. Assess pt for s/s of hair loss
		3. Assess pt's response and use of coping strategies
B. 1. Extravasation will be avoided 2. Skin will heal completely if extravasation occurs	B.	1. Careful technique is used during venipuncture
		2. Administer vesicant through freely flowing IV, constantly monitoring IV site and pt response
		3. Nurse should be *thoroughly* familiar with institutional policy and procedure for administration of a vesicant agent

Vinorelbine *Continued*

Nursing Diagnosis	Defining Characteristics
B. Extravasation	
C. Injection site reactions	C. Erythema and pain at injection site, vein discoloration (33%), mostly mild or moderate; chemical phlebitis proximal to injection site may occur in 10% of pts

Expected Outcomes	**Nursing Interventions**
	4. If vesicant drug is administered as a continuous infusion, drug must be given through a patent central line
	5. If extravasation is suspected:
	a. Stop drug administered
	b. Aspirate any residual drug and blood from IV tubing, IV catheter/needle, and IV site if possible
	c. If drug infiltration is suspected, manufacturer suggests the following after withdrawing any remaining drug from IV: local installation of hyaluronidase, apply moderate heat
	6. Assess site regularly for pain, progression of rythema, induration, and evidence of necrosis
	7. When in doubt whether drug is infiltrating, *treat as an infiltration*
	8. Teach pt to assess site and notify MD if condition worsens
	9. Arrange next clinic visit for assessment of site depending on drug, amount infiltrated, extent of potential injury, and pt variables
	10. Document in pt's record as per institutional policy and procedure
C. 1. Skin changes will be identified early	C. 1. Select vein carefully and alternate venipuncture sites
2. Skin changes will be minimal	2. Consider central access (i.e., VAD) early if pt has limited venous access

Vinorelbine *Continued*

Nursing Diagnosis	Defining Characteristics
C. Injection site reactions	
V. *Potential for sexual/ reproductive dysfunction*	V. A. Drug is teratogenic and fetotoxic

BIBLIOGRAPHY

Abratt, R. P., Bezwoda, W. R., Falkson, G., Goedhals, L., Hacking, D., & Rugg, T. A. (1994). Efficacy and safety profile of gemcitabine in non-small cell lung cancer: a phase II study. *Journal of Clinical Oncology, 12*(8) 1535–1540.

Agarwal, R. (1980). Deoxycoformycin toxicity in mice after long-term treatment. *Cancer Chemotherapy and Pharmacology, 5*(2), 83–87.

Alza Corporation. (2000). VIADUR (leuprolide acetate implant) Healthcare Professional Product Information (pp. 1–10). Mountain View, CA: Alza Corporation.

Amrein, P. C., Davis, R. B., Mayer, R. J., & Schiffer, C. A. (1990). Treatment of relapsed and refractory acute myeloid leukemia with diaziquone and mitoxantrone: A CALGB phase I study. *American Journal of Hematology 35*(2), 80–83.

Anderson, H., Lund, B., Bach, F., Thatcher, N., Walling, J., & Hansen, H. H. (1994). Single-agent activity of weekly gemcitabine in advanced non-small cell lung cancer: A phase II study. *Journal of Clinical Oncology, 12*(9) 1821–1826.

Annual report to the FDA. (1985). CBDCA (NSC #241-240). Washington, DC Government Printing Office.

Beck, S., & Yasko, J. M. (1984). *A guideline for oral care.* Sage Products.

Expected Outcomes	Nursing Interventions
	3. Flush vein after drug administration with at least 75–125 ml of IV solution
V. A. Pt and significant other will identify strategies to cope with altered sexual and reproductive pattern	V. A. As appropriate, explore with pt and significant other issues of reproductive and sexuality pattern and anticipated impact chemotherapy may have B. Counsel female pts of childbearing age in contraceptive options

Becker, T. (1981). *Cancer chemotherapy: A manual for nurses.* Boston: Little, Brown.

Brager, B. L., & Yasko, J. M. (1984). *Care of the client receiving chemotherapy.* Reston, VA: Reston Publishing Co.

Cadman, E. D., Ignoffo, R. J., & Stagg, R. J. (1985). *Leucovorin: Uses with methotrexate, sequential methotrexate and 5-fluorouracil, and with 5-fluorouracil.* Wayne, NJ: Lederle Laboratories.

Calvert, A. H., Harland, J. J., Newell, D. R., et al. (1985). Phase 1 studies with carboplatin at the Royal Marsden Hospital. *Cancer Treatment Review, 12* (suppl A), 54.

Canetta, R., Franks, C., Smaldone, L., et al. (1987, July). Clinical status of carboplatin. *Oncology,* 61–69.

Carella, A. M., Santini, G., Martinengo, M., Giordano, D., Nati, S., Congiu, A., Cerri, R., Risso, M., Damasio, E., & Rossi, E. (1985). 4-demethoxydaunorubicin (Idarubicin) in refractory or relapsed acute leukemia: A pilot study. *Cancer, 55*(7), 1452.

Carter, S. K., Canetta, R., & Roxencweig, M. (1985). Carboplatin: future directions. *Cancer Treatment Review, 12* (suppl A), 145.

Chabner, B. A., & Myers, C. E. (1985). Clinical pharmacology of cancer chemotherapy. In V. T. DeVita, Jr., S. Hellman, & S. A. Rosenberg (Eds.), *Cancer: Principles and practice of oncology* (2nd ed.). Philadelphia: Lippincott.

Daghestani, A. N., et al. (1985). Phase 1–2 clinical and pharmacological study of 4-demethoxydaunorubicin (DMDR) in adult patients with acute leukemia. *Cancer Research, 45*(3), 1408–1412.

Doria, M. I., Shepart, K. V., Lerin, B., & Riddell, R. H. (1986). Liver pathology following hepatic arterial infusion chemotherapy: hepatic toxicity with FUDR. *Cancer, 58*(4), 855–861.

Dorr, R. T. (1989). *MESNEX (Mesna) injection dosing and administration guide—Rationale and guidelines for dosing and administration.* Evansville, IN: Bristol-Myers.

Dorr, R. T., & Fritz, W. (1980). *Cancer chemotherapy handbook.* New York: Elsevier.

Dorr, R. T., & Von Hoff, D. D. (1994). *Cancer chemotherapy handbook* (2nd ed.) Norwalk, CT: Appleton and Lange.

Eisenhower, E. A., Zee, B. C., Pater, J. L., et al. (1988). Trimetrexate: Predictors of severe or life-threatening toxic effects. *Journal of the National Cancer Institute, 80*(16), 1318–1322.

Fischer, D. S., & Knobf, M. T. (1989). *The cancer chemotherapy handbook* (3rd ed.). Chicago: Yearbook Medical Publishers.

Forastiere, A. A., Natale, R. B., Takasugi, B. J., Goren, M. P., Vogel, W. C., & Kudla-Hatch, V. (1987). A phase I–II trial of carboplatin and 5-fluorouracil combination chemotherapy in advanced carcinoma of the head and neck *Journal of Clinical Oncology, 5*(2), 191.

Foster, B. J., Clagett-Carr, K., Leyland-Jones, B., et al. (1985). Results of NCI sponsored phase I trials with carboplatin. *Cancer Treatment Review, 1.* (suppl A), 43.

Goodman, M. (1988). Concepts of hormonal manipulation in the treatment of cancer. *Oncology Nursing Forum, 15*(5), 639–647.

———. (1987). Management of nausea and vomiting induced by outpatient cisplatin therapy. *Seminars in Oncology Nursing, 3* (suppl 1), 23–35.

Govani, L. E., & Hayes, J. E. (1982). *Drugs and nursing implications.* Norwalk CT: Appleton-Century-Crofts.

Grem, J. L., Ellenberg, S.S, King, S. A., et al. (1989). Correlates of severe or life-threatening toxic effects from trimetrexate. *Journal of the National Cancer Institute, 80*(16): 1313–1318.

Grever, M. R., Malspers, L., Balcerzak, S., et al. (1982). 2'-deoxycoformycin A phase I clinical-pharmacokinetic investigation. *AACR Proceedings 23*(533), 36.

Grever, M. R., Siaw, M. F., Jacob, W. F., Neidhart, J. A., Miser, J. S., Coleman, M. S., Hutton, J. J., & Balcerzak, S. P. (1981). The biochemical and clinical consequences of 2'-deoxycoformycin in refractory lymphoproliferative malignancies. *Blood, 57*(2), 406–417.

Grochow, L. B., Noe, D. A., Dole, G. B., & Yarbro, C. H. (1989). Phase I trial of trimetrexate gluconate on a five-day bolus schedule: Clinical pharmacology and pharmacodynamics. *Journal of the National Cancer Institute, 81,* 124–130.

Groenwald, S. L., Frogge, M. H., Goodman, M., & Yarbro, C. H. (1990). *Cancer nursing principles and practice* (2nd ed.). Boston: Jones & Bartlett.

Harris, J. R., Hellman, S., Canellos, G. P., et al. (1985). Cancer of the breast. In V. T. DeVita, Jr., S. Hellman, & S. A. Rosenberg (Eds.), *Cancer: Principles and practice of oncology* (2nd ed.). Philadelphia: Lippincott.

Holmes, F. A., Hwee-Yong, Y. A. P., Esparza, L., Buzdar, A. U., Blumenchein, G. R., Hug, V., & Hortobagyi, G. N. (1987). Mitoxantrone, cyclophosphamide, and fluorouracil in metastatic breast cancer unresponsive to hormonal therapy. *Cancer, 59*(12), 1992–1999.

Hubbard, S. M., & Seipp, C. (1985). Administration of cancer treatments: Practical guide for physicians and oncology nurses. In V. T. DeVita, Jr., S. Hellman, & S. A. Rosenberg (Eds.), *Cancer: Principles and practice of oncology* (2nd ed.). Philadelphia: Lippincott.

Hudes, G. R., & Comis, R. L. (1988). Phase I and II studies of trimetrexate administered in combination with fluorouracil to patients with metastatic cancer. *Seminars in Oncology, 15* (suppl 2), 41–45.

Johnson, B. L., & Gross, J. (1985). *Handbook of oncology nursing.* New York: John Wiley and Sons.

Kemeny, N., Daly, J., Reichman, B., Geller, N., Botet, J., & Odermany, P. (1987). Intrahepatic or systemic infusion of fluorodeoxyuridine in patients with liver metastases from colorectal carcinoma. *Annals of Internal Medicine, 107*(4), 459–465.

Knight, W. A. III, Livingston, R. B., Fabian, C., & Costanzi, J. (1979). Phase I–II trial of methyl-GAG: A SWOG pilot. *Cancer Treatment Report, 63*(11–12), 1933.

Knobf, M. K. T., Fischer, D. S., & Welch-McCaffrey, D. (1984). *Cancer chemotherapy: Treatment and care* (2nd ed.). Boston: G. K. Hall Medical Publishers.

Koeller, J. M., Earhart, R. H., Davis, T. E., et al. (1983). Phase I trial of CBDCA (NSC #241-240) by bolus intravenous injection. *AACR Proceedings, 24*(642), 162 (abstract).

Kris, M. G., D'Acquisto, R. W., Gralla, R. J., Burke, M. T., Marks, L. D., Fanucci, M. P., & Heelan, R. T. (1989). Phase II trial of trimetrexate in patients with stage III and IV non-small cell lung cancer. *American Journal of Clinical Oncology, 12*(1), 24–26.

Kufe, D., Major, P., Agarwal, R., et al. (1980). Phase I–II trial of deoxycoformycin (DCF) in T-cell malignancies. *AACR Proceedings, 21*, 328.

Lambertenghi-Deleliers, G., Pogliani, E., Maiolo, A. T., et al. (1983). Therapeutic activity of 4-demethoxydaunorubicin (DMDR) in adult leukemia. *TUMORI, 69*, 515–519.

Lasley, K., & Ignoffo, R. J. (1981). *Manual of oncology therapeutics.* St. Louis: Mosby.

Lederle Laboratories. (1988). *Novantrone formulary brochure.* Wayne, NJ: Author.

Lee, E. J., Paciucci, A., Amrein, P., et al. (1990). A randomized phase II trial of 3 regimens in the treatment of relapsed or refractory acute myeloid leukemia (AML) in adults: A CALGB study. *ASH Abstracts*, 294a.

Lee, E. J., Van Echo, D. A., Egorin, M. J., Nayar, M. S., Schulman, P., & Schiffer, C. A. (1986). Diaziquone given as a continuous infusion is an active agent for relapsed adult acute nonlymphocytic leukemia. *Blood, 67*(1), 182–187.

Ligha, S. S., Gutterman, J. V., Hall, S. W., et al. (1978). Phase I clinical investigation of 4'-(9-acidinyl-amino) methanesulfon-m-aniside (NSC 249992), a new acridine derivative. *Cancer Research, 38*(11), 3712–3716.

Lu, K., Savaraj, J., Kavanaugh, J., et al. (1984). Clinical pharmacology of 4-demethoxydauno-rubicin. *ASCO Proceedings, 3*(C-147), 88 (abstract).

MacElveen-Hoehn, P. (1985). Sexual assessment and counselling. *Seminar in Oncology Nursing, 1*(1): 69–75.

Major, P. P., Agarwal, R. P., & Kufe, D. W. (1981). Clinical pharmacology of deoxycoformycin. *Blood, 58*(1), 91–96.

Malspers, L., Weinrib, A. B., Staubus, A. E., et al. (1984). Clinical pharmacokinetics of 2'-deoxycoformycin. *Cancer Treatment Symposium, 2*, 7–15.

Marsh, K. C., Liesman, J., Patton, T. F., Fabian, C. J., & Sternson, L. A. (1981). Plasma levels and urinary excretion of methyl-GAG following IV infusion in man. *Cancer Treatment Reports, 65*(3–4), 253.

Mead Johnson Oncology Products. (1989). *The introduction of Ifex and Mesna.* Evansville, IN: Author.

Melmon, K. L., & Morelli, H. F. (1978). *Clinical pharmacology: Basic principles in therapeutics* (2nd ed.). New York: Macmillan.

Micetrick, K. C., Barnes, D., & Erickson, L. C. (1985). A comparison of the cytotoxicity and DNA damaging effects of carboplatin and cisplatin (II). *AACR Proceedings, 26*(1036), 263 (abstract).

Micromedex. (2000). Epirubicin hydrochloride. Web reference: Martindale/Micromedex.

Moertel, R. J. (1990). Does adjuvant therapy work in colon cancer? *New England Journal of Medicine, 322,* 399–401.

Moore, J. O., Schiffer, C. A., Amrein, P., et al. (1992). G-CSF reduces the duration of both granulo-cytopenia and thrombocytopenia after AZQ/mitoxantrone consolidation in acute myelogenous leukemia—CALGB 9022. *ASH Abstracts,* 291a.

Nichols, C., Williams, S., Tricot, G., et al. (1988). Phase I study of high dose etoposide plus carboplatin with autologous bone marrow rescue (ABMT) in refractory germ cell cancer. *ASCO Proceedings, 7*(454), 118 (abstract).

Orphan Medical, Inc. (1999). Busulfex (busulfan) injection: Product monograph. Minnetonka, MN: Orphan Medical.

Paciarini, A., et al. (1983). Pharmacokinetic studies of IV and oral 4-demethoxydaunorubicin in man. *13th International Congress of Chemotherapy.* Vienna, Austria.

Patt, Y. Z., Boddie, A. W., Charnsangavej, C., Ajani, J. A., Wallace, S., Soski, M., Claghorn, L., & Mavligit, G. M. (1986). Hepatic arterial infusion with floxuridine and cisplatin: Overriding importance of antitumor effect vs. degree of tumor burden as determinants of survival among patients with colorectal cancer. *Journal of Clinical Oncology, 4*(9), 1356–1364.

Pazdur, R., Coia, L. R., Hoskins, W. J., et al. (2000). *Cancer management: A multidisciplinary approach* (4th ed.). Melville, NY: PRR.

Perry, M. C., & Yarbro, J. W. (1984). *Toxicity of chemotherapy.* New York: Grune and Stratton.

Peters, F. T. M., Beijnen, J. H., & ten Bokkel Huinink, W. W. (1987). Mitoxantrone extravasation injury. *Cancer Treatment Reports, 71*(10), 992–993.

Physician's Desk Reference. (1986). *Physician's desk reference* (40th ed.). Oradell, NJ: Medical Economics Company, Inc.

————. (2000). 54th ed. Montvale, NJ: Medical Economics Company.

Pratt, W. B., & Ruddon, R. W. (1979). *The anticancer drugs*. New York: Oxford University Press.

Rodrigues, V., Cabanillas, F., Bodey, G. P., et al. (1982). Studies with ifosfamide in patients with malignant lymphoma. *Seminars in Oncology,* (suppl 1), 87.

Schiffer, C. A., Davis, R. B., Mayer, R. J., Peterson, B. A., & Lee, E. J. (1987). Combination chemotherapy with diaziquone and amsacrine in relapsed and refractory acute nonlymphocytic leukemia: A CALGB study. *Cancer Treatment Reports, 71*(9), 879–880.

Silver, R. T., Lauper, R. D., & Jarowski, C. I. (1987). *A synopsis of cancer chemotherapy* (2nd ed.). New York: Yorke Medical Books.

Skeel, R. T. (Ed.). (1982). *Manual of cancer chemotherapy*. Boston: Little, Brown.

Skidmore-Roth, L. (1989). *Mosby's 1989 nursing drug reference*. St. Louis: Mosby.

Smith, I. E., Evans, B. D., Gore, M. E., et al. (1987). Carboplatin (Paraplatin, JMB) and etoposide (VP-16) as first line combination therapy for small cell lung cancer. *Journal of Clinical Oncology, 5*(2), 186.

Solimando, D. A., Bressler, L. R., Kintzel, P. E., & Geraci, M. C. (2000). *Drug information handbook for oncology* (2nd ed.). Cleveland, OH: Lexi-Comp, Inc.

Stewart, J. A., McCormack, J. J., Tong, W., Low, J. B., Roberts, J. D., Blow, A., Whitfield, L. R., Haugh, L. D., Grove, W. R., & Lopez, A. J. (1988). Phase I clinical and pharmacokinetic study of trimetrexate using a daily × 5 schedule. *Cancer Research, 48*(17), 5029–5035.

Tamassia, V., Goldaniga, R., Moroma, A., et al. (1983, December 14–17). Pharmacokinetic studies on three new anthracyclines: Epirubicin, DMDR, esorubicin. *Fourth NCI-EORTC symposium in New Drugs in Cancer Therapy,* 16 (abstract).

Tenebaum, L. (1989). *Cancer chemotherapy: A reference guide.* Philadelphia: W.B. Saunders.

Trissel, L. A., Xu, Q., Kwan, J., & Martinez, J. F. (1994). Compatibility of paclitaxel injection vehicle with IV administration and extension sets. *American Journal of Hospital Pharmacy, 51*(24), 2809–2810

U.S. Department of Health and Human Services. (1989). *National Cancer Institute investigational drugs—Pharmaceutical data 1988* (NIH Publication No. 89-2141). Washington, DC: Author.

von Hoff, D. D. (1987). Whether carboplatin? A replacement for or an alternative to cisplatin. *Journal of Clinical Oncology, 5*(2), 169.

Warrell, R. P., & Burchenal, J. H. (1983). Methyl glyoxal-bis-(Guanylhydrazone) (methyl-GAG): Current status and future prospects. *Journal of Clinical Oncology, 1*(2), 54.

Warrell, R. P., Lee, B. J., Kempin, S. J., Lacher, M. J., Straus, D. J., & Young, C.W. (1981a). Effectiveness of methyl-GAG (methyl glyoxal-bis-[guanylhydrazone]) in patients with advanced malignant lymphoma. *Blood, 57*(6), 1011.

———. (1981b). Clinical evaluation of methyl-GAG (methyl glyoxal-bis-[guanylhydrazone]) alone and in combination with VM-26 (Teniposide), in advanced malignant lymphoma. *AACR and ASCO Proceedings, 22,* 521.

Whitacre, M. Y., & Finley, R. S. (1989). *Paraplatin administration guide.* Evansville, IN: Bristol-Myers Co.

Wilkes, G. M., Ingwersen, K., & Barton-Burke, M. (1993). *Oncology nursing drug reference.* Boston: Jones & Bartlett.

Wilkes, G. M., Ingwersen, K., & Barton-Burke, M. (2000). *2001 oncology nursing drug handbook.* Sudbury, MA: Jones & Bartlett.

Yarbro, C. H. (1989). Carboplatin: A clinical review. *Seminars in Oncology Nursing, 5* (suppl 1), 63–69.

Appendices

APPENDIX 1

Chemotherapy Checklist and Nursing Guidelines

APPENDIX 2

Extravasation

APPENDIX 3

Hypersensitivity and Anaphylactic Reactions

APPENDIX 4

Illustrated Guide to Handling Cytotoxic and Hazardous Drugs

Appendix 1

Chemotherapy Checklist and Nursing Guidelines

Appendix 1.1   Multidisciplinary Practice Guidelines

I. Baseline professional training

   A. Three primary disciplines are involved in the chemotherapy process. Each professional should have a baseline knowledge of cancer chemotherapy before practicing.

      1. Physicians authorized to write chemotherapy orders for neoplastic disease states should be board-certified and/or board-eligible hematologists or medical, pediatric, radiation (for specified drugs on protocol), or gynecologic oncologists and the oncology fellows who have been deemed capable by the section chief. An attending physician thus qualified should routinely check and countersign chemotherapy orders written by an oncology fellow during the first two months on the clinical service.

      2. In acute-care hospitals that are not solely cancer centers, many non-oncology specialties use antineoplastic drugs for treatment of non-malignant conditions in dermatology (e.g., methotrexate for psoriasis) or rheumatology (cyclophosphamide for patients with lupus nephritis). The recommendations for these non-oncology specialties that use cytotoxic chemotherapy include having the department or section register with the pharmacy department the usual agents, dose ranges, and indicated diseases, with provision of published reference sources and/or institutional review board-approved protocols for these treatments.

      3. Registered nurses who will handle and administer chemotherapy need to be cancer chemotherapy-certified. Certification includes:
         • attending a chemotherapy certification course
         • successful completion of a written examination
         • demonstrated competency in administering chemotherapy
         • attendance at a yearly update session to remain certified

      4. Pharmacists involved in chemotherapy practice must complete the departmental staff development chemotherapy lecture series. Completion includes:
         • successful completion of a written examination
         • demonstrated competency in safe and accurate chemotherapy compounding and handling
         • attendance at a yearly update session to remain certified

II. Standard practice

   A. Oncologists or oncology fellows should be solely responsible for writing chemotherapy orders and/or entering them into a computer or specially authorized chemotherapy order form. To maintain a system of checks, it is imperative that the physicians complete the first step of order-writing, which includes dose calculations and modifications. This also encompasses a practice of limiting verbal chemotherapy orders to dose reduction in modification of an existing order.

B. The chemotherapy order should be composed in a standard format. Computer order sets should be created and/or order sheets preprinted with standard and commonly used regimens. Drugs should always be ordered by the generic or U.S. Assigned Name, consistent with usage in the hospital formulary, and the three federally recognized compendia. Although the trade name or an abbreviation or jargon name may be placed in parentheses if it will add to the clarity of the order, it is not an acceptable substitute for the generic name even though a cooperative group protocol uses it. When free-form chemotherapy orders are written for unusual or nonstandard drug regimens, a reference to the source(s) that provided the basis for the order must be cited and, when possible, a copy of the relevant source placed in the chart and an explanation given in writing as to why this particular therapy was chosen. Initial creation of preprinted orders or order sets should be the responsibility of one discipline and verified independently by the other two. This would include a formal sign-off when the check is complete.

C. Journal articles, abstracts, outside institutional protocols, and any other potential treatment references that represent the source of the orders or clarify them should be made known to all involved professionals by placement of a direct copy in the patient's chart before treatment. Copies of outside institutional protocols should also be made available to the pharmacist. This direct copy should contain at least the following information: generic drug name, dose, dosage schedule, side effects or toxicity, rationale for the regimen, necessary dose reductions, and administration guidelines.

D. All orders should be written using the following format: generic drug name, dose to be given (in milligrams), dosage used (milligrams per meter squared or per kilogram), frequency, days of administration, and infusion guidelines. Ordinarily, the total dose for the course should not be listed on the order sheet or the computer order screen, lest it be misinterpreted as a single dose to be administered. (For continuous infusion pump delivery, the total dose to be infused over the set period must be included, but there should be a notation of how much is to be delivered each day.) All pertinent information must be supplied to ensure a safe and accurate order capable of verification.

E. Standard chemotherapy reference texts and handbooks and standard drug references should be readily available to physicians, nurses, and pharmacists on all patient-care areas and the central and decentralized pharmacy.

F. An increasing number of patients are being treated on protocols. Any protocol that accrues patients must be approved by the institutional review board. When a new protocol is instituted, multidisciplinary education must take place before patient enrollment. This is especially important when protocols involve investigational agents, high-dose therapy, and unusual or new combination therapies. This education must ensure adequate communication between the principle investigator, clinic nurses, research nurses, inpatient nurses, and all oncology pharmacists. Copies of all new protocols and amendments must be placed in designated patient-care areas, clinics, and central and decentralized pharmacies. Preprinted or computer order sets should be configured and in place before patient enrollment to avoid order variability and ambiguity. New protocols or unusual therapies should not begin off-hours or on weekends unless it is an acute emergency situation. They should be initiated on weekdays when appropriate specialists and clinicians are available.

G. Order verification and/or double-checking enhances safe chemotherapy practice, and there should not be any exceptions to this. The nurse and pharmacist are each independently responsible for the following:

- check entire order set against an acceptable reference (protocol, journal article, chemotherapy text or handbook, abstract, computer hard copy of order set, etc.)
- verify that current body surface area, height, and weight are correct
- verify the final dose of each drug
- check the rate of administration, amount, and type of solution
- check the antiemetic regimen, prehydration and posthydration, for omissions or additions of ancillary medication therapy
- compare current orders with previous therapy—consider any radical changes
- check that an X-ray has been read to confirm central venous access for new line placements for continuous vesicant infusions
- if dose modification has been made, confirm parameters with reference or research protocol and then consult with prescriber to verify rationale if nonstandard modification was made
- determine if appropriate laboratory values are within normal parameters, based on known organ-specific toxicity of each drug, in addition to hematologic parameters; abnormal values should be called to the attention of the prescriber and treatment modifications made after adequate discussion

The nursing verification should be completed by two nurses, one of whom is a certified chemotherapy nurse. Each should sign each chemotherapy order. Nurses must also verify availability of progenitor cells with attending oncologist or oncology fellows in situations that involve bone marrow transplant or stem cell transplant. Research nurses are also responsible for checking laboratory parameters dictated by the research protocol. In addition to the above expectations for pharmacy, pharmacists must ensure that the prescribed solution and administration parameters will enable adequate drug delivery and ensure compatibility of chemotherapy with intravenous solutions and/or additives. Once orders are double-checked, they should be prepared and labeled following pharmacy compounding policies and safe handling procedures.

H. Chemotherapy administration may begin once the final product, which has been checked by a pharmacist, arrives in the designated patient care area. Two nurses, one of whom must be chemotherapy-certified, must check the final product against the original order before administration. In the clinic setting, one certified nurse and pharmacist should check the final product before administration. The check should take place at the patient's bedside so that the two professionals can ensure that the correct drug is being given to the appropriate patient by checking the identification band in the same fashion that a blood transfusion is checked. The attending oncologist and/or oncology fellow may also administer chemotherapy when necessary after following comparable procedures.

I.   Chemotherapy administration should occur on dedicated oncology inpatient units and ambulatory oncology sites that are staffed by certified chemotherapy nurses. On occasion, patients are on other units or must be transferred, such as a patient on continuous infusion to an intensive care unit. That nursing staff should then be educated by a certified chemotherapy nurse. All oncology settings should have a standard oncology text, chemotherapy handbook, copies of approved protocols, and a standard drug reference.

J.   The attending physician who writes the chemotherapy order should be required to include the cumulative dose of anthracycline, bleomycin, and mitomycin previously received by the patient. It should be noted that the system instituted to require notation of previously received cumulative doses should not require current dose and previous dose to be noted on the same screen or together as part of the order, to avoid confusion and potential error.

Source: Fischer, D. S., Alfano, S., Knobf, M. T., Donovan, C., and Beaulieu, N. (1996). Improving the cancer chemotherapy use process. *Journal of Clinical Oncology, 14*(12), 3148–3155. Reprinted with permission.

Appendix 1.2 Prechemotherapy Nursing Assessment Guidelines

Potential Problems/ Nursing Diagnoses	Physical Status: Assessment Parameters/ Signs and Symptoms
Hematopoietic system	
A. Impaired tissue perfusion related to chemotherapy-induced anemia	• Hgb g (norms 12–14; 14–16) • Hct% (norms 32–36; 36–40) • Vital signs (BP, pulse, respiration) • Pallor (face, palms, conjunctiva) • Fatigue or weakness • Vertigo
B. Impaired immunocompetence and potential for infection related to chemotherapy-induced leukopenia	• WBC (norm 4500–9000/mm³) • Pyrexia/rigor, erythema, swelling, pain any site) • Abnormal discharges, draining wounds, skin/mucous membrane lesions • Productive cough, SOB, rectal pain, urinary frequency
C. Potential for injury (bleeding) related to chemotherapy-induced thrombocytopenia	• Platelet count (150,000–400,000/mm³) • Spontaneous gingival bleeding or epistaxis • Presence of petechiae or easy bruisability • Hematuria, melena, hematemesis, hemoptysis • Hypermenorrhea • S/s of intracranial bleeding (irritability, sensory loss, unequal pupils, headache, ataxis)
Integumentary system	
Alteration in mucous membrane of mouth, nasopharynx, esophagus, rectum, anus, or ostomy stoma related to chemotherapy-induced tissue changes	Mucositis Scale 0 = pink, moist, intact mucosa; absence of pain or burning + 1 = generalized erythema with or without pain or burning + 2 = isolated small ulcerations and/or white patches + 3 = confluent ulcerations with white patches on 25% mucosa + 4 = hemorrhagic ulcerations

Drug- and Dose-Limiting Factors

- Hgb < 8 g
- Hct < 20%
- Blood transfusions not initiated

- WBC < 3,000/mm^3
- Fever > 101°F
  —Hold all myelosuppressive agents (exceptions may include leukemia, lymphoma, and/or situations in which there is neoplastic marrow infiltration)

- Platelet count < 100,000/mm^3
  —Hold all myelosuppressive agents (exceptions may include leukemia, lymphoma, and/or situations in which there is neoplastic marrow infiltration)

- + 2 mucositis
  — Hold antimetabolites (esp. methotrexate, 5-FU)
  — Hold antitumor antibiotics (esp. doxorubicin, dactinomycin)

Appendix 1.2 *Continued*

Potential Problems/ Nursing Diagnoses	Physical Status: Assessment Parameters/ Signs and Symptoms
Gastrointestinal system	
Discomfort, nutritional deficiency, and/or fluid and electrolyte disturbances related to chemotherapy-induced:	
A. Anorexia	• Lab values: albumin and total protein • Normal weight/present weight and % of body weight loss • Normal diet pattern/changes in diet pattern • Alterations in taste sensation • Early satiety
B. Nausea and vomiting	• Lab values: electrolytes • Pattern of nausea/vomiting (incidence, duration, severity) • Antiemetic plan Drug(s), dosage(s), schedule, efficacy • Other (dietary adjustments, relaxation techniques, environmental manipulation)
C. Bowel disturbances	
1. Diarrhea	• Normal pattern of bowel elimination • Consistency (loose, watery/bloody stools) • Frequency and duration (#/day and # of days) • Antidiarrheal drug(s), dosage(s), efficacy
2. Constipation	• Normal pattern of bowel elimination • Consistency (hard, dry, small stools) • Frequency (hours or days beyond normal pattern) • Stool softener(s), laxative(s), efficacy

Drug- and Dose-Limiting Factors

- Intractable nausea/vomiting × 24 hrs if IV hydration not initiated

- Diarrheal stools × 3 per 24 hrs
  —Hold antimetabolites (esp. methotrexate, 5-FU)
- No BM × 48 hrs past normal bowel patterns
  —Hold vinca alkaloids (vinblastine, vincristine)

Appendix 1.2 *Continued*

Potential Problems/ Nursing Diagnoses	Physical Status: Assessment Parameters/ Signs and Symptoms
D. Hepatotoxicity	• Lab values: LDH, SGOT, alk phos, bilirubin • Pain/tenderness over liver, feeling of fullness • Increase in nausea/vomiting or anorexia • Changes in mental status • Jaundice • High-risk factors —Hepatic metastasis —Viral hepatitis —Abdominal XRT —Concurrent hepatotoxic drugs —Graft vs. host disease —Blood transfusions
Respiratory system Impaired gas exchange or ineffective breathing pattern related to chemotherapy-induced pulmonary fibrosis	• Lab values: PFTs, CXR • Respiration (rate, rhythm, depth) • Chest pain • Nonproductive cough • Progressive dyspnea • Wheezing/stridor • High-risk factors —Total cumulative dose of bleomycin —Preexisting lung disease —Prior/concomitant XRT —Age > 60 yrs —Concomitant use of other pulmonary toxic drugs —Smoking hx
Cardiovascular system Decreased cardiac output related to chemotherapy-induced: A. Cardiac arrhythmias B. Cardiomyopathy	• Lab values: cardiac enzymes, electrolytes, EKG, ECHO, MUGA • Vital signs • Presence of arrhythmia (irregular radial/apical) • S/s of CHF (dyspnea, ankle edema, nonproductive cough, rales, cyanosis) • Hold anthracyclines • High-risk factors —Total cumulative dose anthracyclines —Preexisting cardiac disease —Prior/concurrent mediastinal XRT —Bolus administration higher drug doses

Drug- and Dose-Limiting Factors

- Evidence of chemical hepatitis
  —Hold hepatotoxic agents (esp. methotrexate, 6-MP) until differential dx established

- Acute unexplained onset respiratory symptoms
  —Hold all antineoplastic agents until differential dx established

- Acute s/s of CHF and/or cardiac arrhythmia
  —Hold all antineoplastic agents until differential dx established
- Total dose doxorubicin or daunorubicin > 550 mg/m^2

Appendix 1.2 *Continued*

Potential Problems/ Nursing Diagnoses	Physical Status: Assessment Parameters/ Signs and Symptoms
Genitourinary system	

A. Alteration in fluid volume (excess) related to chemotherapy-induced:
  1. Glomerular or renal tubule damage
  2. Hyperuricemic nephropathy
B. Alteration in comfort related to chemotherapy-induced hemorrhagic cystitis
	• Lab values: BUN, creatinine clearance, serum creatinine, uric acid, electrolytes, urinalysis
	• Color, odor, clarity of urine
	• 24-hr fluid I&O (estimate/actual)
	• Hematuria; proteinuria
	• Development of oliguria or anuria
	• High-risk factors
	  —Preexisting renal disease
	  —Concurrent treatment with nephrotoxic drugs (esp. aminoglycoside antibiotics)

Nervous system	

A. Impaired sensory/motor function related to chemotherapy-induced:
  1. Peripheral neuropathy
  2. Cranial nerve neuropathy
 	
B. Impaired bowel and bladder elimination related to chemotherapy-induced autonomic nerve dysfunction
	• Paresthesias (numbness, tingling in feet, fingertips)
	• Trigeminal nerve toxicity (severe jaw pain)
	• Diminished or absent deep tendon reflexes (ankle and knee jerks)
	• Motor weakness, slapping gait, ataxia
	• Visual and auditory disturbances
	• Urinary retention
	• Constipation, abdominal cramping and distention
	• High-risk factors
	  —Changes in diet or mobility
	  —Frequent use of narcotic analgesics
	  —Obstructive disease process

Source: Adapted from Engelking, C. (1988). Prechemotherapy nursing assessment in outpatient settings. *Outpatient Chemotherapy, 3*(1), 9–11. Reprinted with permission from World Health Communications, Inc.

**Drug- and Dose-Limiting
Factors**

- Hematuria
  —Hold cyclophosphamide serum creatinine > 2.0 and/or creatinine
    clearance < 70 ml/min
  —Hold Cis-platinum, streptozocin anuria × 24 hrs
  —Hold all antineoplastic agents

- Presence of any neurologic s/s
  —Hold vinca alkaloids, Cis-platinum, hexamethylmelamine, procarbazine
    until differential dx established
- Presence of any neurologic s/s
  —Hold vinca alkaloids until differential dx established

Appendix 1.3   Chemotherapy Checklist

1. Verify informed consent: may be written or oral depending on institution policy, but it is required before chemotherapy administration.

2. Know the drug pharmacology: mechanism of action; usual dosage; route of administration; acute and long-term side effects; and route of excretion.

3. Review laboratory data keeping in mind acceptable parameters. Report abnormalities to the physician.

4. Complete prechemotherapy assessment of patient, medical history, and prior chemotherapy.

5. Check physician order for name of drug(s): dosage; route; rate; and timing of drug(s) administration. (Question anything that seems out of the ordinary.)

6. Recalculate dosage: check height and weight; calculate body surface area (BSA).

7. Verify physician orders and dosage calculations with another nurse.

8. Premedication: administer most premedications at least 20–30 minutes before chemotherapy starts. In some cases, may want to start the patient on antiemetic therapy the night before or the morning of therapy.

9. Patient education: teach and review with the patient and family details of the chemotherapy schedule, expected side effects, and self-care preventive management suggestions to minimize untoward side effects. Provide written explanations the patient can refer to later because this information may be overwhelming. Refer questions to physician as necessary.

10. Provide patient with telephone numbers for physician and clinic, as appropriate.

11. Reconstitute drug(s) according to manufacturer suggestions, OSHA guidelines, and institution procedures. May be the responsibility of the nursing or the pharmacy department, depending on the institution's policy.

12. Gather appropriate equipment: D_5W or normal saline (NS) are commonly used to infuse chemotherapy, but not exclusively. Use the correct solution and volume. Protect from direct sunlight if applicable.

13. Administer chemotherapy agents according to written policies and procedures using proficient intravenous therapy skills and techniques.
    a. Administer all medications using the five rights:
       (1) Right Patient
       (2) Right Drug
       (3) Right Dose
       (4) Right Route
       (5) Right Time
    b. If no information is available, assume the drug you are giving is a vesicant and administer it with caution, according to institutional policy and procedure.
    c. Avoid drug infiltration: if unsure whether the IV is infiltrated, discontinue it, and restart another IV rather than risk extravasation. WHEN IN DOUBT, PULL IT OUT.
    d. Do not mix drugs together when administering combination therapy. Use syringe or intravenous of NS to flush before first drug, in between drugs, and upon completion of all drugs.
    e. It is not optimal to administer vesicant drugs through an indwelling peripheral IV (one that has been in place 4–6 hours or more). It is important to preserve veins, but it is more important to prevent potential extravasation.
    f. Nonvesicant chemotherapy drugs may be administered through an existing IV, once the site has been fully assessed for patency and lack of infiltration.
    g. If unable to start an IV after two attempts, consult a colleague for assistance.
14. Do not allow anyone to interrupt you during the preparation or administration of chemotherapy.
15. Do not foster a patient's dependency on one nurse.
16. Always have emergency drugs and an extravasation kit readily available should an adverse reaction occur.

17. Always listen to the patient: the patient's knowledge and preference should be utilized as frequently as possible. As the patient becomes more knowledgeable regarding IV techniques, his or her personal experience with successful IV sites, methods, and sensations can be a great aid to the nurse. Even at times when the patient's preference may not be the best choice, his or her participation should always be encouraged.

18. Dispose of intravenous supplies according to OSHA guidelines, and institution policy and procedure.

19. Document drug administration according to institution policy and procedures. Use time savers in documentation, e.g., instead of writing step-by-step how a vesicant was given, write "(Name of drug) administered according to institution policy and procedure for vesicants."

20. Observe for adverse reactions.

21. Use the opportunity to teach and counsel the patient and the family while administering the chemotherapy.

Sources: Oncology Nursing Society. (1988). *Cancer Chemotherapy Guidelines: Module II. Recommendations for Nursing Practice in the Acute Care Setting.* Pittsburgh: Oncology Nursing Society Press; Morra, M. E. (ed). (1981). *Cancer Chemotherapy Treatment and Care.* Boston: G. K. Hall Medical; Miller, S. A. (1980). Nursing actions in cancer chemotherapy administration. *Oncology Nursing Forum,* 7(4), 8–16.

Appendix 2

Extravasation

Appendix 2.1   Vesicants and Irritants

Vesicants		
Chemotherapeutic Agents	**Antidote**	**Antidote Preparation**
Alkylating agents		
mechlorethamine hydrochloride (nitrogen mustard)	Isotonic sodium (Na) thiosulfate	Prepare 1/6 molar solution: a. If 10% Na thiosulfate solution, mix 4 ml with 6 ml sterile water for injection b. If 25% Na thiosulfate solution, mix 1.6 ml with 8.4 ml sterile water
cisplatin (Platinol[a])	Same as above	Same as above
Antitumor antibiotics		
doxorubicin (Adriamycin[b])	None	
daunorubicin (Cerubidine[c])	None	
mitomycin-C (Mitomycin)	None	
dactinomycin (Actinomycin-D)	None	

Vesicants

Local Care	Comments
1. Immediately inject Na thiosulfate through IV cannula, 2 ml for every mg extravasated 2. Remove needle 3. Inject antidote into subcutaneous (SC) tissue	1. Na thiosulfate neutralizes nitrogen mustard, which then is excreted via the kidneys 2. Time is essential in treating extravasation 3. Heat and cold not proven effective 4. Although clinically accepted, reports of the benefits are scant
1. Use 2 ml of the 10% Na thiosulfate for each 100 mg of cisplatin 2. Remove needle 3. Inject SC	1. Vesicant potential seen with a concentration of more than 20 cc of 0.5 mg/ml extravasates. If less than this, drug is an irritant; no treatment recommended
1. Apply cold pad with circulating ice water, ice pack, or cryogel pack for 15–20 minutes at least four times per day for the first 24–48 hours	1. Extravasations of less than 1–2 cc often will heal spontaneously; if greater than 3 cc, ulceration often results 2. Protect from sunlight and heat 3. Studies suggest benefit of 99% dimethyl sulfoxide (DMSO) 1–2 ml applied to site every six hours (Olver et al. 1988; St. Germain, Houlihan, and D'Amato 1994). Other studies show delayed healing with DMSO
	1. Little information known 2. In mouse experiments, some benefit from topical DMSO
	1. Protect from sunlight 2. Delayed skin reactions have occurred in areas far from original IV site 3. Some research studies show benefit with use of 99% DMSO 1–2 ml applied to site every six hrs for 14 days. More studies needed
1. Apply ice to increase comfort at the site 2. Elevate for 48 hrs then resume normal activity	1. Heat may enhance tissue damage

Appendix 2.1 *Continued*

Vesicants		
Chemotherapeutic Agents	**Antidote**	**Antidote Preparation**
mitoxantrone	Unknown	
epirubicin Idarubicin (Idamycin[d]) esorubicin	None	
Vinca alkaloids/ microtubular inhibiting agents vincristine (Oncovin[e])	hyaluronidase*	Mix 150 units hyaluronidase with 1–3 ml saline
vinblastine (Velban[e])	Same as above	Same as above
vindesine	Same as above	Same as above
vinorelbine (Navelbine[f])	Same as above	Same as above
Taxanes paclitaxel (Taxol[a])	hyaluronidase* Ice	

Vesicants	
Local Care	**Comments**
	1. Antidote or local care measures unknown 2. Ulceration rare unless concentrated dose infiltrates
	1. Antidote and local care measures unknown 2. Cold, DMSO, and corticosteroids ineffective in experiments with mice. Esorubicin-phlebitis common
1. Apply warm pack for 15–20 mins at least 4 times per day for the first 24–48 hrs and elevate Same as above Same as above Same as above	1. Administer hyaluronidase and apply heat for 15–20 mins at least 4 times per day for the first 24–48 hrs 2. These two methods of treatment are very effective for rapid absorption of drug Same as above Same as above 1. Same treatment as vincristine/vinblastine 2. Moderate vesicant 3. Manufacturer recommends administering drug over 6–10 mins into side port of freeflowing IV closest to the IV bag, followed by flush of 75–125 ml of IV solution to reduce incidence of phlebitis and severe back pain
1. Apply ice pack for 15–20 mins at least 4 times per day for the first 24 hrs	1. Recent documentation of vesicant potential 2. Paclitaxel has rare vesicant potential (probably due to dilution in 500 cc diluent) 3. Ice and hyaluronidase have been effective in decreasing local tissue damage in a mouse model

Appendix 2.1 *Continued*

Irritants		
Chemotherapeutic Agents	**Antidote**	**Antidote Preparation**
Alkylating agents dacarbazine (DTIC)		
ifosfamide carboplatin		
Nitrosoureas carmustine (BCNU)		
Antitumor antibiotics doxorubicin liposome		
bleomycin		
menogaril		
Vinca alkaloids etoposide (VP-16)	hyaluronidase*	
teniposide (VM-26)		

[a] Bristol-Myers Squibb Oncology, Princeton, NJ; [b]Pharmacia & Upjohn Co., Kalamazoo, MI; [c] Chiron Therapeutics, Emeryville, CA; [d] Adria Laboratories, Dublin, OH; [e] Eli Lilly and Co. Indianapolis, IN; [f] Glaxo Wellcome Oncology/HIV, Research Triangle Park, NC

* Hyaluronidase is no longer manufactured.

Note: Based on information from Bertelli, G., et al. (1995). Topical dimethylsulfoxide for the prevention of soft tissue injury after extravasation of vesicant cytotoxic drugs: A prospective clinical study. *Journal of Clinical Oncology, 13*(11), 2851–2855; Lebredo, L., Barrie, R., and

	Irritants	
Local Care	**Comments**	
	1. May cause phlebitis 2. Protect from sunlight 1. May cause phlebitis 2. Antidote or local care measures unknown	
	1. May cause phlebitis 2. Antidote or local care measures unknown	
	1. May produce redness and tissue edema 2. Low ulceration potential 3. If ulceration begins or pain, redness, or swelling persist, treat like doxorubicin 1. May cause irritation to tissue 2. Little information known 1. May cause phlebitis, venous edema, and induration 2. Increased incidence if concentrations greater than 1 mg/ml infiltrates or administration occurs in more than 2 hours	
1. Apply warm pack	1. Treatment necessary only if large amount of a concentrated solution extravasates. In this case, treat like vincristine or vinblastine 2. May cause phlebitis, urticaria, and redness Same as above	

Woltering, E. A. (1992). DMSO protection against adriamycin-induced tissue necrosis. *Journal of Surgery Research, 53*(1), 26–65; Rospond, E. M., and Engel, L. M. (1993). Dimethyl sulfoxide for treating anthracycline extravasation. *Clinical Pharmatherapeutics, 12*(8), 560–561.

Source: Oncology Nursing Society. (1999). *Cancer Chemotherapy Guidelines and Recommendations for Practice* (2nd ed.). Pittsburgh: Oncology Nursing Society Press. Reprinted with permission.

Appendix 2.2   Standardized Nursing Care Plan for Patients Experiencing Extravasation

Nursing Diagnosis	Defining Characteristics
I. *Potential alteration in skin integrity related to extravasation*	I. Vesicant drugs may cause erythema, burning, tissue necrosis, tissue sloughing
II. *Potential pain at site of extravasation*	II. Vesicant drugs include A. Commercial agents 　1. dactinomycin 　2. daunorubicin 　3. doxorubicin 　4. mitomycin C 　5. mechlorethamine 　6. vinblastine 　7. vincristine 　8. vinorelbine 　9. idarubicin 　10. vindesine 　11. epirubicin 　12. esorubicin 　13. cisplatin 　14. mitoxantrone 　15. paclitaxel B. Investigational agents 　1. amsacrine 　2. maytansine 　3. bisantrene 　4. pyrazofurin 　5. adozelesin 　6. anti-B4-blocked ricin

Expected Outcomes	Nursing Interventions
I. Extravasation, if it occurs, will be detected early with early intervention	I. Careful technique is used during venipuncture A. Select venipuncture site away from underlying tendons and blood vessels. B. Secure IV so that catheter/needle site is visible at all times. C. Administer vesicant through freely flowing IV, constantly monitoring IV site and pt response. Nurse should be thoroughly familiar with institutional policy and procedure for administration of a vesicant agent. D. If vesicant drug is administered as a continuous infusion, drug must be given through a patent central line.
II. Skin and underlying tissue damage will be minimized	II. If extravasation is suspected: A. Stop drug administration. B. Aspirate any residual drug and blood from IV tubing, IV catheter/needle, and IV site if possible. C. Instill antidote if one exists through needle if able to remove remaining drug in previous step. If standing orders are not available, notify MD and obtain order. D. Remove needle. E. Inject antidote into area of apparent infiltration if antidote is recommended, using 25-gauge needle into subcutaneous tissue. F. Apply topical cream if recommended. G. Cover lightly with occlusive sterile dressing. H. Apply warm or cold applications as prescribed. I. Elevate arm. J. Assess site regularly for pain, progression of erythema, induration, and evidence of necrosis:

Appendix 2.2   *Continued*

Nursing Diagnosis	Defining Characteristics
III. *Potential loss of function of extremity related to extravasation*	
IV. *Potential infection related to skin breakdown*	

Source: Berg, D. (1996). Principles of chemotherapy administration. In
M. Barton-Burke, G. Wilkes, and K. Ingwersen, *Cancer Chemotherapy: A Nursing Process Approach* (2nd ed.). Sudbury, MA: Jones & Bartlett.

Expected Outcomes	Nursing Interventions
	1. If outpatient, arrange to assess site or teach pt to and to notify provider if condition worsens. Arrange next visit for assessment of site depending on drug, amount infiltrated, extent of potential injury, and pt variables.
	2. Discuss with MD the need for plastic-surgical consult if erythema, induration, pain, tissue breakdown occurs.
	K. When in doubt about whether drug is infiltrating, treat as an infiltration.
	L. Document precise, concise information in patient's chart.
	1. Date, time
	2. Insertion site, needle size and type
	3. Drug administration technique, drug sequence, and approximate amount of drug extravasated
	4. Appearance of site, patient's subjective response
	5. Nursing interventions performed to manage extravasation, and notification of MD
	6. Photo documentation if possible
	7. Follow-up plan
	8. Nurse's signature
	9. Institutional policy and procedure for documentation should be adhered to

Appendix 2.3   Nursing Assessment of Extravasation Versus Other Reactions

Assessment Parameter	Extravasation	
	Immediate Manifestations	**Delayed Manifestations**
Pain	Severe pain or burning that lasts minutes or hours and eventually subsides; usually occurs while the drug is being given and around the needle site	Hours–48
Redness	Blotchy redness around the needle site; not always present at time of extravasation	Later occurrence
Ulceration	Develops insidiously; usually occurs 48–96 hours later	Later occurrence
Swelling	Severe swelling; usually occurs immediately	Hours–48
Blood return	Inability to obtain blood return	Good blood return during drug administration
Other	Change in the quality of infusion	Local tingling and sensory deficits

Source: Oncology Nursing Society. (1999). *Cancer Chemotherapy Guidelines and Recommendations for Practice* (2nd ed.). Pittsburgh: Oncology Nursing Society Press. Reprinted with permission.

Irritation of the Vein	Flare Reaction
Aching and tightness along the vein	No pain
The full length of the vein may be reddened or darkened.	Immediate blotches or streaks along the vein, which usually subside within 30 minutes with or without treatment
Not usually	Not usually
Not likely	Not likely; wheals may appear along vein line
Usually	Usually
	Uritcaria

Appendix 3

Hypersensitivity and Anaphylactic Reactions

Appendix 3.1   Types of Hypersensitivity Reactions (Gell and Coombs Classification)

Type	Major Signs and Symptoms	Example of Reaction	Mechanism of Action
I	Anaphylactic symptoms: urticaria, angioedema, rash, bronchospasm, abdominal cramping, respiratory collapse, and cardiovascular collapse	Anaphylaxis to chemotherapy, bee stings, food allergies	IgE-mediated HSR; antigen-IgE antibody interaction on basophil and mast cell surfaces causing degranulation
II	Hemolytic anemia, cardiovascular collapse, and possibly death	Massive hemolysis from transfusion of incompatible blood	Cell surface antigens interacting with IgG or IgM antibodies with destruction (lysis) of target cell
III	Deposition of immune complexes in tissues resulting in various forms of tissue injury and manifestations	Systemic lupus, rheumatoid arthritis, horse serum sickness; may produce a maculopapular eruption or vasculitic lesions	Antigen-antibody interaction, forming immune complexes; anaphylactoid reaction from complement activation via classical pathway, may mimic type I reaction
IV	Stomatitis, pneumonitis, contact dermatitis, granuloma formation, and homograft rejection	Tuberculosis, poison ivy, contact sensitivity from mechlorethamine topical application for mycosis fungoides	Sensitized T lymphocytes react with antigen and release lymphokines

Source: Labovich, T. M. (1999). Acute hypersensitivity reactions to chemotherapy. *Seminars in Oncology Nursing, 11*(3), 225. Reprinted with permission.

Appendix 3.2   Summary of Chemotherapy Agents With a
                High Incidence of Hypersensitivity Reactions

Drug	Factors Increasing Risk of HSRs	Comments
L-asparaginase	Administered as a single agent After fourth dose	HSR most likely IgE-mediated *Erwinia* asparaginase can be substituted if reaction occurs
	Hiatus of > 1 month between doses Weekly administration versus daily or 3×/week Prior exposure to L-asparaginase, months or even years previously Intravenous route of administration High doses	Pegasparaginase under investigation as a substitute
paclitaxel	Faster infusion rate Higher dosage	Premedication with dexamethasone, diphenhydramine, HCl, and cimetadine, famotadine, or ranitadine ± ephedrine to prevent reaction
etoposide		Can occur with the first dose or subsequent doses
teniposide		HSR can occur shortly after or several hours after infusion No published reports of HSR to oral etoposide
cisplatin	Six or more doses Intravesicular route of administration*	HSRs are less common now compared with their initial use; may be attributed to fewer

Appendix 3.2   *Continued*

Drug	Factors Increasing Risk of HSRs	Comments
		courses and current trends of antiemetic use with diphenhydramine and dexamethasone
		Cross-reactivity exists between carboplatin and cisplatin
procarbazine		Pulmonary toxicity has been reported in anecdotal form
melphalan and chlorambucil	At least 2 prior doses of melphalan	Chlorambucil has a few type I reactions with urticaria and angioedema but no hypotension
anthracycline antibiotics	Intravesical administration of doxorubicin	Flare reactions usually do not progress to acute HSR[†]
		Sudden cardiac arrest during infusion, although rare, is considered a direct cardiac toxicity versus an acute HSR
cyclophosphamide and ifosfamide		Can occur with both oral and intravenous administration
		Mesna also has been reported to cause type I HSRs

*Intravesicular administration typically has a higher number of courses of treatment; premedication for nausea and vomiting is not needed as with intravenous administration.
[†]Acute HSR involves serum sickness, bronchospasm, parental medication administration, and/or anaphylaxis.

Source: Labovich, T. M. (1999). Acute hypersensitivity reactions to chemotherapy. *Seminars in Oncology Nursing, 11*(3), 224. Reprinted with permission.

Appendix 3.3 Management of Hypersensitivity and Anaphylactic Reactions

1. Review the pt's allergy history.
2. Consider prophylactic medications with hydrocortisone or an antihistamine in atopic/allergic individuals (this requires a physician's order).
3. Pt and family education: Assess the pt's readiness to learn. Inform pt of the potential of an allergic reaction and report any unusual symptoms such as:
   a. Uneasiness or agitation
   b. Abdominal cramping
   c. Itching
   d. Chest tightness
   e. Lightheadedness or dizziness
   f. Chills
4. Ensure emergency equipment and medications are readily available.
5. Obtain baseline vital signs and note pt's mental status.
6. As appropriate, perform a scratch test, intradermal skin test, or test dose before administering the full dosage (this requires a physician's order). If there is no reaction, the remaining dose can be administered. If an allergic response is suspected, discontinue the test dose (unless it has been completed), maintain the intravenous line, and notify the physician.
7. For a localized allergic response:
   a. Evaluate symptoms; observe for urticaria, wheals, localized erythema.
   b. Administer diphenhydramine or hydrocortisone as per physician's order.
   c. Monitor vital signs every 15 minutes for 1 hour.
   d. Continue subsequent dosing or desensitization program according to a physician's order.
   e. If a "flare" reaction appears along the vein with doxorubicin (Adriamycin) or daunorubicin, flush the line with saline.
      (1) Ensure that extravasation has not occurred.
      (2) Administer hydrocortisone 25–50 mg intravenously with a physician's order followed by a normal saline flush. This may be adequate to resolve the "flare" reaction.
      (3) After the "flare" reaction has resolved, continue slow infusion of the drug.
      (4) Monitor for repeated "flare" episodes. It is preferable to change the intravenous site if possible.
8. For a generalized allergic response, anaphylaxis may be suspected if the following signs or symptoms occur (usually within the first 15 minutes of the start of the infusion or injection):
   a. Subjective signs and symptoms
      (1) Generalized itching

Appendix 3.3 *Continued*

      (2) Chest tightness

      (3) Difficulty speaking

      (4) Agitation

      (5) Uneasiness

      (6) Dizziness

      (7) Nausea

      (8) Crampy abdominal pain

      (9) Anxiety

     (10) Sense of impending doom

     (11) Desire to urinate or defecate

     (12) Chills

  b. Objective signs

      (1) Flushed appearance (edema of face, hands, or feet)

      (2) Localized or generalized urticaria

      (3) Respiratory distress with or without wheezing

      (4) Hypotension

      (5) Cyanosis

9. For a generalized allergic response:

  a. Stop the infusion immediately and notify the physician.

  b. Maintain the intravenous line with appropriate solution to expand the vascular space, e.g., normal saline.

  c. If not contraindicated, ensure maximum rate of infusion if the pt is hypotensive.

  d. Position the pt to promote perfusion of the vital organs; the supine position is preferred.

  e. Monitor vital signs every 2 minutes until stable, then every 5 minutes for 30 minutes, then every 15 minutes as ordered.

  f. Reassure the pt and the family.

  g. Maintain the airway and anticipate the need for cardiopulmonary resuscitation.

  h. All medications must be administered with a physician's order.

10. Document the incident in the medical record according to institutional policy and procedures.

11. Physician-guided desensitization may be necessary for subsequent dosing.

Source: Berg, D. (1996). Principles of chemotherapy administration. In M. Barton-Burke, G. Wilkes, and K. Ingwersen. *Cancer Chemotherapy: A Nursing Process Approach.* Sudbury, MA: Jones & Bartlett. Reprinted with permission.

Appendix 3.4 Standardized Nursing Care Plan for Patient Experiencing Hypersensitivity or Anaphylaxis

Nursing Diagnosis	Defining Characteristics
I. *Potential for injury related to hypersensitivity or anaphylaxis*	I. A. Allergic or hypersensitivity reactions to chemotherapy vary from simple allergic reactions to life-threatening ones B. The reactions are the result of a foreign substance being introduced into the body, with resultant antibody formation C. The reactions may worsen with subsequent exposure to the foreign substance (chemotherapeutic agent)

Expected Outcomes	**Nursing Interventions**

I. A. Allergic reactions (hypersensitivity and anaphylaxis), if they occur, will be detected early
B. Airway will remain patent
C. BP will remain within 20 mmHg of baseline
D. Future allergic responses will be prevented
	I. A. Review standing orders for management of allergic reactions (hypersensitivity and anaphylaxis) per institutional policy and procedure
	B. Identify location of anaphylaxis kit; the kit should contain:
	  1. epinephrine 1:1000
	  2. hydrocortisone sodium succinate (SoluCortef)
	  3. diphenhydramine HCl (Benadryl)
	  4. aminophylline
	  5. similar emergency drugs
	C. Prior to drug administration, obtain baseline vital signs and record mental status
	D. Observe for following s/s, usually occurring within the first 15 mins of infusion
	  1. *Subjective*
	    a. nausea
	    b. generalized itching
	    c. crampy abdominal pain
	    d. chest tightness
	    e. anxiety
	    f. agitation
	    g. sense of impending doom
	    h. wheeziness/shortness of breath
	    i. desire to urinate/defecate
	    j. dizziness
	    k. chills
	  2. *Objective*
	    a. flushed appearance (angioedema of the face, neck, eyelids, hands, feet)
	    b. localized or generalized urticaria
	    c. respiratory distress and wheezing
	    d. hypotension
	    e. cyanosis

Appendix 3.4 *Continued*

Nursing Diagnosis	Defining Characteristics

Source: Berg, D. (1996). Principles of chemotherapy administration. In M. Barton-Burke, G. Wilkes, and K. Ingwersen, *Cancer Chemotherapy: A Nursing Process Approach.* Sudbury, MA: Jones & Bartlett.

Expected Outcomes	Nursing Interventions
	E. ONS recommendations for generalized allergic response
	1. Stop infusion and notify MD
	2. Obtain orders for infusion of NS to maintain vascular volume and titrate infusion rate to maintain adequate BP (i.e., within 20 mmHG of baseline systolic BP)
	3. Place pt in supine position to promote perfusion of visceral organs
	4. Monitor vital signs q 2 mins until stable, then q 5 mins for 30 mins, then q 15 mins
	5. Provide emotional reassurance to pt and family
	6. Maintain patent airway and have equipment ready for CPR if needed
	7. Medications per MD order and institutional policy and procedure
	F. Document incident
	G. Discuss with MD desensitization versus drug discontinuance for further dose

Appendix 4

Illustrated Guide to Handling Cytotoxic and Hazardous Drugs

This reference chart is designed to provide basic information regarding the safe handling of widely used cytotoxic and hazardous drugs. It is intended to supplement the knowledge of physicians, nurses, pharmacists, and other health care professionals regarding the safe handling of drugs used in clinical practice.

This information is advisory only and is not intended to replace sound clinical judgment in the delivery of health care services. For access to more detailed information, please refer to the list of references provided. Please consult complete prescribing information for any drug mentioned herein.

GUIDELINES FOR HANDLING SPILLS AND ACCIDENTS

Spill Kits

- Spill kit should include:
1. Two pairs disposable latex, vinyl, or nitrile gloves; utility gloves
2. Low-permeability, disposable protective garments (coveralls or closed-front gown and shoe covers)
3. Safety glasses or splash goggles

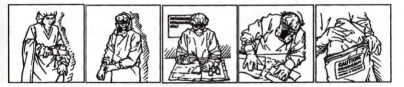

4. NIOSH*-approved respirator (when a spill presents risk of inhalation of airborne powder or aerosol)
5. Absorbent, plastic-backed sheets and spill pads
6. Disposable toweling
7. At least two sealable thick plastic hazardous-waste disposable bags (prelabeled with an appropriate warning label)
8. A disposable scoop for collecting glass fragments
9. A puncture-resistant container for glass fragments

*National Institute of Occupational Safety and Health

General Procedures

- "Spill kits" containing all of the materials needed to clean up spills of hazardous drugs should be available in all areas where hazardous drugs are routinely handled
- Wearing protective apparel from the spill kit, workers should remove any broken glass fragments and place them in the puncture-resistant container
- For spills involving no breakage, use absorbent pads or sponges
- Clean all spill areas three times with a detergent solution, followed by water
- Limit access to the contaminated area until cleanup is complete

Cleanup of Small Spills (<5 ml or 5 g)

- Wear gown, double gloves, and eye protection
- Use absorbent gauze pads for cleanup of liquids; use damp gauze pads for solids

Cleanup of Large Spills (>5 ml or 5 g)

- Wear gown, double gloves, and eye protection
- Use NIOSH-approved respirator if airborne particles or aerosols are likely to be present during cleanup
- Starting from the edge of the spill, use absorbent sheets, spill pads, or spill pillows for cleanup of liquids; use damp cloths or towels for solids

In Case of Contamination of Personnel

- Remove contaminated gloves or garments immediately

- Wash hands after removing gloves (some drugs are known to penetrate gloves)
- In case of skin contact with a hazardous drug, thoroughly wash the affected area with soap and water; seek medical attention if appropriate
- In case of eye exposure, flush affected eye with copious amounts of water or eye-flush kit, as directed; seek medical attention if appropriate
- Refer to preestablished policies and procedures for personnel contamination

---

RISKS OF EXPOSURE TO CYTOTOXIC AND HAZARDOUS DRUGS

Primary Routes of Exposure
- Trauma (needle sticks, etc.)
- Inhalation of drug aerosols or droplets
- Absorption through direct skin contact

Procedures that Pose Risk of Exposure During Drug Preparation
- Withdrawal of needles from vials
- Drug transfers using syringes or needles
- Opening ampules
- Expulsion of air from drug-filled syringe
- Changing IV bottles or IV tubing
- Priming IV tubing
- Breakage of vials, IV bottles, etc.

Procedures that Pose Risk of Exposure During Drug Administration
- Clearing air from a syringe or IV tubing (e.g., priming IV tubing)
- Accidental puncture of a closed system
- Leakage from tubing, syringe, or connection site
- Clipping needles

Procedures that Pose Risk of Exposure During Disposal of Contaminated Material

- Handling body fluids (blood, excreta, vomitus, ascitic fluid, pleural fluid) of patients who are receiving cytotoxic and hazardous drugs
- Disposal of linens or other materials soaked with body fluids
- Handling spills of cytotoxic and hazardous drugs

RECOMMENDED EQUIPMENT AND PREPARATION AREA FOR HANDLING CYTOTOXIC AND HAZARDOUS DRUGS

Gloves

- Permeability of glove material varies with the drug, contact time, and glove thickness; thicker material reduces risk of exposure
- Recommended: thicker, longer, powder-free, disposable latex, vinyl, or nitrile gloves or glove liners
- Two pairs of fresh gloves should be put on when beginning any task or batch and changed hourly or immediately if they are torn, punctured, or contaminated with a spill
- Wash hands before and after gloving

  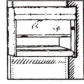

Non-Absorbent, Disposable Gown

- Recommended design: Non-absorbent, disposable, lint-free gown of low-permeability fabric with closed front and long sleeves with elastic or knit cuffs
- Gown should be worn during drug preparation, administration, and waste disposal
- Avoid use of open-front lab coats or nondisposable gowns

Class II or III Vertical Laminar Airflow Biological Safety Cabinet (BSC)

- A vertical laminar airflow BSC is preferred to a horizontal airflow workstation

- Meets National Sanitation Foundation (NSF) Standard 49
- The BSC should be on at all times (24 hours a day, 7 days a week)
- The BSC should be placed in a draft-free area that is not subject to frequent personnel traffic since front opening of unit still presents potential for contamination and exposure
- The BSC should be decontaminated on a regular basis (ideally at least weekly) and whenever there is a spill or the BSC is moved or serviced

Goggles

- Plastic face shield or splash goggles complying with American National Standards Institute (ANSI)

Working Inside a BSC

- Vertical laminar airflow Class II or III biological safety cabinet
- Disposable plastic-backed paper liner for work surface

Working without a BSC is not Recommended

PREPARATION AND ADMINISTRATION TECHNIQUES

Before Handling Syringes, IV Bottles, Bags, Ampules, or Vials

- Double gloving is recommended when beginning any task or batch
- Change outer glove immediately whenever contamination occurs
- Thoroughly wash and dry hands before gloves are donned and when a task or batch is completed

Handling Syringes, Needles, and IV Bottles/Bags

- Use proper aseptic technique
- Properly label all syringes, IV bags, and bottles according to guidelines of institution/facility
- Syringes should be large enough so that they are not full when containing the total drug dose
- Attach and prime drug administration sets within the BSC before drug is added to fluid

- Dispose of used syringes and needles in a puncture-proof container designed for hazardous chemical waste disposal without crushing, clipping, or capping

Handling Vials

- Avoid venting medication vials unless using venting devices such as filter needles or dispensing pins
- Use Luer-lock type syringe and needle fittings
- Add diluent slowly to the vial by alternately injecting small amounts, allowing air to be displaced
- Maintain negative pressure while withdrawing drug from vial

Handling Ampules

- Tap down any material remaining in the neck and top of an ampule before opening
- Wrap sterile gauze pad around ampule neck before breaking the top
- Keep ampule away from face while opening top
- If diluent is to be added, inject diluent slowly down the inside wall of ampule
- Tap ampule gently to ensure that all powder is wet before agitating to dissolve contents

Work Practices

- Wash hands before putting on gloves
- Change gowns or gloves immediately if they become contaminated
- Watch infusion sets and pumps for signs of leakage during use; place a plastic-backed absorbent pad under tubing during use to catch any leakage
- Prime the administration set in a BSC using a sterile gauze pad; if priming at site of administration, the IV line should be primed with nondrug-containing fluid or a backflow closed system should be used

- Do not crush or clip used needles and syringes; place in a hazardous chemical waste container
- After administration of drug, place all gauze and alcohol wipes into a hazardous chemical waste container; wash hands upon removal of gloves

---

SAFETY ISSUES AND WASTE DISPOSAL

Policies and Procedures

- Establish and maintain written policies and procedures for handling cytotoxic and hazardous drugs
- Address personnel issues of conception, pregnancy, and breast-feeding in all these policies and procedures
- Include a list of cytotoxic and hazardous drugs in the policies and procedures
- Make policies and procedures easily and readily available to all personnel expected to handle cytotoxic and hazardous drugs
- Make information available on toxicity, treatment of acute exposure, chemical inactivators, solubility, and stability of cytotoxic and hazardous drugs used in the institution/facility

Training and Supervision

- Orientation and training should include:
  —discussion of known and potential hazards of cytotoxic and hazardous drugs
  —explanation of all relevant policies
  —techniques and procedures
  —proper use of protective equipment and materials
- Contents of orientation program and attendance should be well documented and meet "worker right to know" statutes and regulations

Verification and Documentation of Compliance

- Knowledge and competence of personnel preparing and administering cytotoxic and hazardous drugs should be evaluated after initial training and at regular intervals
- Evaluation should include written examination and observed demonstration of competence in preparation and simulated administration of practice solutions

- All personnel involved with cytotoxic and hazardous drugs should be continually updated on new or revised information on safe handling of these drugs

Supplies and Handling

- All health-care workers who handle cytotoxic and hazardous drugs or waste must be oriented to and must follow procedures governing the identification, containment, collection, segregation, and disposal of cytotoxic and hazardous drug waste materials
- Handle hazardous chemical waste containers with uncontaminated gloves
- Store hazardous chemical waste in labeled, leakproof drums or cartons (in accordance with state and local regulations and disposal contractor's requirements) at a designated area until disposal

 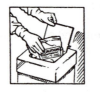

Disposal

- All hazardous chemical waste must be segregated from all other trash
- Hazardous chemical waste from drug preparation and patient-care areas should be disposed of as hazardous or toxic waste in an EPA-permitted, state-licensed hazardous-waste incinerator
- Comply with applicable federal, state, and local regulations regarding disposal

PHYSICAL INTEGRITY AND SECURITY OF CYTOTOXIC AND HAZARDOUS DRUG SUPPLIES

Limited Access Storage/Work Area

- Access to storage/work area for cytotoxic and hazardous drugs should be limited to specified personnel
- For storage of cytotoxic and hazardous drugs, use shelves, bins, carts, counters, and trays designed to avoid falling and breakage

- Store cytotoxic and hazardous drugs requiring refrigeration separately from other drugs, in individual bins designed to prevent breakage and contain leakage

Handling Damaged Goods

- Maintain written procedures for handling damaged packages of cytotoxic and hazardous drugs; train shipping and receiving personnel in these procedures, including proper use of protective garments and equipment
- Receive and open damaged goods in an isolated area or BSC

Identify Drugs that Require Special Handling

- Establish list of cytotoxic and hazardous drugs that require special handling, and post in appropriate locations
- Place appropriate warning labels on all cytotoxic and hazardous drug cartons, shelves, and bins where the drug products are stored

Commonly Used Cytotoxic and Hazardous Drugs

altretamine	carboplatin	cisplatin
aminoglutethimide	carmustine	cyclophosphamide
azathioprine	chlorambucil	cyclosporin
L-asparaginase	chloramphenicol	cytarabine
bleomycin	chlorotrianisene	dacarbazine
busulfan	chlorozotocin	dactinomycin

daunorubicin
diethylstilbestrol
doxorubicin
estradiol
estramustine
ethinyl estradiol
etoposide
floxuridine
fluorouracil
flutamide
ganciclovir
hydroxyurea
idarubicin
ifosfamide
interferon-A

isotretinoin
leuprolide
levamisole
lomustine
mechlorethamine
medroxyprogesterone
megestrol
melphalan
mercaptopurine
methotrexate
mitomycin
mitotane
mitoxantrone
nafarelin

pipobroman
plicamycin
procarbazine
ribavirin
streptozocin
tamoxifen
testolactone
thioguanine
thiotepa
uracil mustard
vidarabine
vinblastine
vincristine
zidovudine

Adapted from OSHA (1995) Work-practice guidelines for personnel dealing with cytotoxic (antineoplastic) drugs. Office of Occupational Medicine, Directorate of Technical Support, OSHA, April 14; and Cetus Corporation (1991) Safe handling of cytotoxic and hazardous drugs.

REFERENCES

American Medical Association Council on Scientific Affairs. (1985). Guidelines for handling parenteral antineoplastics. *Journal of the American Medical Association, 253,* 1590–1592.

American National Standards Institute. (1968). Occupational and Educational Eye and Face Protection. *ANSI Z87.1.*

American Society of Hospital Pharmacists. (1990). ASHP technical assistance bulletin on handling cytotoxic and hazardous drugs. *American Journal of Hospital Pharmacology, 47,* 1033–1049.

Andersen, R., Boedicker, M., Ma, M., Goldstein, E. J. (1986). Adverse reactions associated with pentamidine isethionate in AIDS patients: recommendations for monitoring therapy. *Drug Intell. Clin. Pharm.* 20: 862–868.

Anderson, R. W., Puckett, W. H. Jr., Dana, W. J., Nguyen, T. V., Theiss, J. C., & Matney, T. S. (1982). Risk of handling injectable antineoplastic agents. *American Journal of Hospital Pharmacology, 39,* 1881–1887.

Avis, K. E., & Levchuck, J. W. (1984). Special considerations in the use of vertical laminar flow workbenches. *American Journal of Hospital Pharmacology, 41,* 81–87.

Barber, R. K. (1981). Fetal and neonatal effects of cytotoxic agents. *Obstetric Gynecology, 51,* 41S–47S.

Benhamou, S., Pot-Deprun, J., Sancho-Garnier, H., & Chouroulinkov, I. (1988). Sister chromatid exchanges and chromosomal aberrations in lymphocytes of nurses handling cytostatic drugs. *International Journal of Cancer, 41,* 350–353.

Bos, R. P., Leenars, A. O., Theuws, J. L., & Henderson, P. T. (1982). Mutagenicity of urine from nurses handling cytostatic drugs, influence of smoking. *International Archive of Occupational Environmental Health, 50,* 359–369.

Bryan, D., & Marback, R. C. (1984). Laminar-airflow equipment certification: What the pharmacist needs to know. *American Journal of Hospital Pharmacology, 41,* 1343–1349.

Burgaz, S., Ozdamar, Y. N., & Karakaya, A. E. (1988). A signal assay for the detection of genotoxic compounds: Application on the urines of cancer patients on chemotherapy and of nurses handling cytotoxic drugs. *Human Toxicology, 7,* 557–560.

California Department of Health Services Occupational Health Surveillance and Evaluation Program. (1986). *Health care worker exposure to ribavirin aerosol: field investigation FI-86-009.* Berkeley: California Department of Health Services.

Castegnaro, M., Adams, J., & Armour, M. A. (Eds.). (1985). *Laboratory decontamination and destruction of carcinogens in laboratory wastes: Some antineoplastic agents.* International Agency for Research on Cancer. Scientific Publications No. 73. Lyon, France: IARC.

Chapman, R. M. (1984). Effect of cytotoxic therapy on sexuality and gonadal function. In M. C. Perry & J. W. Yarbro (Eds.), *Toxicity of chemotherapy.* Orlando, FL: Grune and Stratton. (pp. 343–363).

Chen, C. H., Vazquez-Padua, M., & Cheng, Y. C. (1990). Effect of antihuman immunodeficiency virus nucleoside analogs on mDNA and its implications for delayed toxicity. *Molecular Pharmacology, 39,* 625–628.

Christensen, C. J., Lemasters, G. K., & Wakeman, M. A. (1990). Work practices and policies of hospital pharmacists preparing antineoplastic agents. *Journal of Occupational Medicine, 32,* 508–512.

Chrysostomou, A., Morley, A. A., & Seshadri, R. (1984). Mutation frequency in nurses and pharmacists working with cytotoxic drugs. *Australia New Zealand Journal of Medicine, 14,* 831–834.

Connor, J. D., Hintz, M., & Van Dyke, R. (1984). Ribavirin pharmacokinetics in children and adults during therapeutic trials. In R. A. Smith, V. Knight, & J. A. D. Smith (Eds.), *Clinical applications of ribavirin.* Orlando, FL: Academic Press.

Connor, T. H., Laidlaw, J. L., Theiss, J. C., Anderson, R. W., & Matney, T. S. (1984). Permeability of latex and polyvinyl chloride gloves to carmustine. *American Journal of Hospital Pharmacology, 41,* 676–679.

Crudi, C. B. (1980). A compounding dilemma: I've kept the drug sterile but have I contaminated myself? *National Intravenous Therapy Journal, 3,* 77–80.

Dole *v.* United Steelworkers, 494 U.S.26. (1990).

Doll, D. C. (1989). Aerosolised pentamidine. *Lancet, ii,* 1284–1285.

Duvall, E., & Baumann, B. (1980). An unusual accident during the administration of chemotherapy. *Cancer Nursing, 3,* 305–306.

Environmental Protection Agency. (1991). *Discarded commercial chemical products, off specification species, container residues, and spill residues thereof.* 40 CFR 261.33(f).

Everson, R. B., Ratcliffe, J. M., Flack, P. M., Hoffman, D. M., & Watanabe, A. S. (1985). Detection of low levels of urinary mutagen excretion by chemotherapy workers which was not related to occupational drug exposure. *Cancer Research, 45,* 6487–6497.

Falck, K., Grohn, P., Sorsa, M., Vainio, H., Heinonen, E., & Holsti, L. R. (1979). Mutagenicity in urine of nurses handling cytostatic drugs. *Lancet, i,* 1250–1251.

Falck, K., Sorsa, M., & Vainio, H. (1981). Use of the bacterial fluctuation test to detect mutagenicity in urine of nurses handling cytostatic drugs (abstract). *Mutation Research, 85,* 236–237.

Ferguson, L. R., Everts, R., Robbie, M. A., et al. (1988). The use within New Zealand of cytogenetic approaches to monitoring of hospital pharmacists for exposure to cytotoxic drugs: Report of a pilot study in Auckland. *Australian Journal of Hospital Pharmacology, 18,* 228–233.

Gude, J. K. (1989). Selective delivery of pentamidine to the lung by aerosol. *American Review of Respiratory Diseases, 139,* 1060.

Guglielmo, B. J., Jacobs, R. A. , & Locksley, R. M. (1989). The exposure of health care workers to ribavirin aerosol. *Journal of the American Medical Association, 261,* 1880–1881.

Harrison, R., Bellows, J., Rempel, D., et al. (1988). Assessing exposures of health-care personnel to aerosols of ribavirin—California. *Morbidity and Mortality Weekly Report, 37,* 560–563.

Hemminki, K., Kyyronen, P., & Lindbohm, M. L. (1985). Spontaneous abortions and malformations in the offspring of nurses exposed to anaesthetic gases, cytostatic drugs, and other potential hazards in hospitals, based on registered information of outcome. *Journal of Epidemiology Community Health, 39,* 141–147.

Henderson, D. K., & Gerberding, J. L. (1989). Prophylactic zidovudine after occupational exposure to the human immunodeficiency virus: an interim analysis. *Journal of Infectious Diseases, 160,* 321–327.

Hillyard, I. W. (1980). The preclinical toxicology and safety of ribavirin. In Smith, R. A., Kirkpatrick, W. (Eds.): *Ribavirin: A broad spectrum antiviral agent.* New York, Academic Press.

Hirst, M., Tse, S., Mills, D. G., Levin, & White, D. F. (1984). Occupational exposure to cyclophosphamide. *Lancet, 1,* 186–188.

Hoy, R. H., & Stump, L. M. (1984). Effect of an air-venting filter device on aerosol production from vials. *American Journal of Hospital Pharmacology, 41,* 324–326.

International Agency for Research on Cancer. (1975). *IARC monographs on the evaluation of the carcinogenic risk of chemicals to man: Some aziridines, N-, S-, and O-mustards and selenium,* Vol. 9. Lyon, France: IARC.

International Agency for Research on Cancer. (1976). *IARC monographs on the evaluation of the carcinogenic risk of chemicals to man: Some naturally occurring substances,* Vol. 10. Lyon, France: IARC.

International Agency for Research on Cancer. (1981). *IARC monographs on the evaluation of the carcinogenic risk of chemicals to humans: Some antineoplastic and immunosuppressive agents,* Vol. 26. Lyon, France: IARC.

International Agency for Research on Cancer. (1982). *IARC monographs on the evaluation of the carcinogenic risk of chemicals to humans: Chemicals, industrial processes and industries associated with cancer in humans,* Vols. 1–29.(suppl 4). Lyon, France: IARC.

International Agency for Research on Cancer. (1987a). *IARC monographs on the Evaluation of the carcinogenic risk of chemicals to humans, Genetic and related effects, An updating of selected IARC monographs from volumes 1–42,* Vols. 1–42 (suppl 6). Lyon, France: IARC

International Agency for Research on Cancer. (1987*b*). *IARC monographs on the evaluation of the carcinogenic risk of chemicals to humans; Overall evaluations of carcinogenicity: An Updating of IARC monographs Volumes 1 to 42*, Vols. 1–42 (suppl 7). Lyon, France: IARC.

International Agency for Research on Cancer. (1990). *IARC monographs on the evaluation of the carcinogenic risk of chemicals to humans: Pharmaceutical drugs*, Vol. 50. Lyon, France: IARC.

Jagun, O., Ryan, M., & Waldron, H. A. (1982). Urinary thioether excretion in nurses handling cytotoxic drugs. *Lancet, i*, 443–444.

Johnson, E. G., & Janosik, J. E. (1989). Manufacturer's recommendations for handling spilled antineoplastic agents. *American Journal of Hospital Pharmacology, 46*, 318–319.

Juma, F. D., Rogers, H. J., Trounce, J. R., & Bradbrook, I. D. (1978). Pharmacokinetics of intravenous cyclophosphamide in man, estimated by gas-liquid chromotography. *Cancer Chemotherapy Pharmacology, 1*, 229–231.

Kacmarek, R. M. (1990). Ribavirin and pentamidine aerosols: Caregiver beware! *Respiratory Care, 35*, 1034–1036.

Karakaya, A. E., Burgaz, S., & Bayhan, A. (1989). The significance of urinary thioethers as indicators of exposure to alkylating agents. *Archives of Toxicology, 13* (suppl), 117–119.

Kilham, L., & Ferm, V. H. (1977). Congenital anomalies induced in hamster embryos with ribavirin. *Science, 195*, 413–414.

Kleinberg, M. L., & Quinn, M. J. (1981). Airborne drug levels in a laminar-flow hood. *American Journal of Hospital Pharmacology, 38*, 1301–1303.

Kolmodin-Hedman, B., Hartvig, P., Sorsa, M., & Falck, K. (1983). Occupational handling of cytostatic drugs. *Archives of Toxicology, 54*, 25–33.

Kyle, R. A. (1984). Second malignancies associated with chemotherapy. In M. C. Perry & J. W. Yarbro (Eds.), *Toxicity of chemotherapy* (pp. 479–506). Orlando, FL: Grune and Stratton.

Laidlaw, J. L., Connor, T. H., Theiss, J. C., Anderson, R. W. & Matney, T. S. (1984). Permeability of latex and polyvinyl chloride gloves to 20 antineoplastic drugs. *American Journal of Hospital Pharmacology, 41*, 2618–2623.

Laidlaw, J. L., Connor, T. H., Theiss, J. C., Anderson, R. W., & Matney, T. S. (1985). Permeability of four disposable protective-clothing materials to seven antineoplastic drugs. *American Journal of Hospital Pharmacology, 42,* 2449–2454.

Lee, S. B. (1988). Ribavirin—exposure to health care workers. *American Ind. Hyg. Association, 49,* A13–14.

LeRoy, M. L., Roberts, M. J. & Theisen, J. A. (1983). Procedures for handling antineoplastic injections in comprehensive cancer centers. *American Journal of Hospital Pharmacology, 40,* 601–603.

Lunn, G., & Sansone, E. B. (1989). Validated methods for handling spilled antineoplastic agents. *American Journal of Hospital Pharmacology, 46,* 1131.

Lunn, G., Sansone, E. B., Andrews, A. W., & Hellwig, L. C. (1989). Degradation and disposal of some antineoplastic drugs. *Journal of Pharmacology Sciences, 78,* 652–659.

Matthews, T., & Boehme, R. (1988). Antiviral activity and mechanism of action of ganciclovir. *Review of Infectious Diseases, 10* (suppl 3), s490–s494.

McDevitt, J. J., Lees, P. S. J., & McDiarmid, M. A. (1993). Exposure of hospital pharmacists and nurses to antineoplastic agents. *Journal of Occupational Medicine, 35,* 57–60.

McDiarmid, M. A., Egan, T., Furio, M., Bonacci, M., & Watts, S. R. (1988). Sampling for airborne fluorouracil in a hospital drug preparation area. *American Journal of Hospital Pharmacology, 43,* 1942–1945.

McDiarmid, M. A., & Emmett, E. A. (1987). Biological monitoring and medical surveillance of workers exposed to antineoplastic agents. *Seminars in Occupational Medicine, 2,* 109–117.

McDiarmid, M. A., & Jacobson-Kram, D. (1989). Aerosolized pentamidine and public health. *Lancet, ii,* 863–864.

McDiarmid, M. A. (1990). Medical surveillance for antineoplastic-drug handlers. *American Journal of Hospital Pharmacology, 47,* 1061–1066.

McDiarmid, M. A., Gurley, H. T., & Arrington, D. (1991). Pharmaceuticals as hospital hazards: Managing the risks. *Journal of Occupational Medicine, 33,* 155–158.

McDiarmid, M. A., Kolodner, K., Humphrey, F., et al. (1992). Baseline and phosphoramide mustard-induced sister-chromatid exchanges in pharmacists handling anti-cancer drugs. *Mutation Research, 279,* 199–204.

McDiarmid, M. A., Schaefer, J., Richard, C. L., Chaisson, R. E. , & Tepper, B. S. (1992). Efficacy of engineering controls in reducing occupational exposure to aerosolized pentamidine. *Chest, 102,* 1764–1766.

McEvoy, G. K. (Ed.). (1993). *American hospital formulary service drug information*. Bethesda, MD: American Society of Hospital Pharmacists.

McLendon, B. F., & Bron, A. F. (1978). Corneal toxicity from vinblastine solution. *British Journal of Ophthalmology, 62*, 97–99.

National Sanitation Foundation. (1990). *Standard No. 49 for class II (laminar flow) biohazard cabinetry.* Ann Arbor, MI: National Sanitation Foundation.

National Study Commission on Cytotoxic Exposure. (1983). *Recommendations for handling cytotoxic agents.* Louis P. Jeffrey, Sc.D., Chairman, Rhode Island Hospital, Providence, Rhode Island.

National Study Commission on Cytotoxic Exposure. (1984). *Consensus responses to unresolved questions concerning cytotoxic agents.* Louis P. Jeffrey, Sc.D., Chairman, Rhode Island Hospital, Providence, Rhode Island.

Neal, A. D., Wadden, R. A., & Chiou, W. L. (1983). Exposure of hospital workers to airborne antineoplastic agents. *American Journal of Hospital Pharmacology, 40*, 597–601.

Nikula, E., Kiviniitty, K., Leisti, J., & Taskinen, P. (1984). Chromosome aberrations in lymphocytes of nurses handling cytostatic agents. *Scandinavian Journal of Work Environmental Health, 10*, 71–74.

Norppa, H., Sorsa, M., Vainio, H., et al. (1980). Increased sister chromatid exchange frequencies in lymphocytes of nurses handling cytostatic drugs. *Scandinavian Journal of Work Environmental Health, 6*, 229–301.

Nguyen, T. V., Theiss, J. C., & Matney, T. S. (1982). Exposure of pharmacy personnel to mutagenic antineoplastic drugs. *Cancer Research, 42*, 4792–4796.

Palmer, R. G., Dore, C. J., & Denman, A. M. (1984). Chlorambucil-induced chromosome damage to human lymphocytes is dose-dependent and cumulative. *Lancet, i*, 246–249.

Perry, M. C., & Yarbro, J. W. (Eds.). (1984). *Toxicity of chemotherapy.* Orlando FL: Grune and Stratton.

Physician's Desk Reference. (1991). *Physician's desk reference* (45th ed. p. 730). Oradell, NJ: Medical Economics Data.

Pohlova, H., Cerna, M., & Rossner, P. (1986). Chromosomal aberrations SCE and urine mutagenicity in workers occupationally exposed to cyto static drugs. *Mutation Research, 174*, 213–217.

Pyy, L., Sorsa, M., & Hakala, E. (1988). Ambient monitoring of cyclophosphamide in manufacture and hospitals. *American Industrial Hygiene Association Journal, 49*, 314–317.

Reich, S. D., & Bachur, N. R. (1975). Contact dermatitis associated with adriamycin (NSC-123127) and daunorubicin (NSC-82151). *Cancer Chemotherapy Reports, 59*, 677–678.

Reynolds, R. D., Ignoffo, R., Lawrence, J., Torti, F. M., Koretz, M., Anson, N., & Meier, A. (1982). Adverse reactions to AMSA in medical personnel. *Cancer Treatment Reports, 66*, 1885.

Rogers, B. (1987). Health hazards to personnel handling antineoplastic agents. *Occupational Medicine: State of the Art Reviews, 2*, 513–524.

Rogers, B., & Emmett, E. A. (1987). Handling antineoplastic agents: Urine mutagenicity in nurses. *IMAGE Journal of Nursing Scholarship, 19*, 108–113.

Rosner, F. (1976). Acute leukemia as a delayed consequence of cancer chemotherapy. *Cancer, 37*, 1033–1036.

Rudolph, R., Suzuki, M,. & Luce, J. K. (1979). Experimental skin necrosis produced by adriamycin. *Cancer Treatment Reports, 63*, 529–537.

Schafer, A. I. (1981). Teratogenic effects of antileukemic therapy. *Archives of Internal Medicine, 141*, 514–515.

Selevan, S. G., Lindbolm, M. L., Hornung, R. W., & Hemminki, K. (1985). A study of occupational exposure to antineoplastic drugs and fetal loss in nurses. *New England Journal of Medicine, 313*, 1173–1178.

Siever, S. M. (1975). Cancer chemotherapeutic agents and carcinogenesis. *Cancer Chemotherapy Reports, 59*, 915–918.

Sieber, S. M., & Adamson, R. H. (1975). Toxicity of antineoplastic agents in man: chromosomal aberrations, antifertility effects, congenital malformations, and carcinogenic potential. *Advanced Cancer Research, 22*, 57–155.

Siebert, D., & Simon, U. (1973). Cyclophosphamide: pilot study of genetically active metabolites in the urine of a treated human patient. *Mutagenic Research, 19*, 65–72.

Slevin, M. L., Ang, L. M., Johnston, A., & Turner, P. (1984). The efficiency of protective gloves used in the handling of cytotoxic drugs. *Cancer Chemotherapy Pharmacology, 12*, 151–153.

Smaldone, G. C., Vincicuerra, C., & Marchese, J. (1991). Detection of inhaled pentamidine in health care workers. *New England Journal of Medicine, 325*, 891–892.

Sorsa, M., Hemminki, K., & Vainio, H. (1985). Occupational exposure to anticancer drugs—potential and real hazards. *Mutation Research, 154*, 135–149.

Sotaniemi, E. A., Sutinen, S., Arranto, A. J., et al. (1983). Liver damage in nurses handling cytostatic agents. *Acata Med. Scand., 214,* 181–189.

Stellman, J. M. (1987). The spread of chemotherapeutic agents at work: Assessment through stimulation. *Cancer Investigation, 5,* 75–81.

Stephens, J. D., Golbus, M. S., Miller, T. R., Wilber, R. R., & Epstein, C. J. (1980). Multiple congenital abnormalities in a fetus exposed to 5-fluorouracil during the first trimester. *American Journal of Obstetrics and Gynecology, 137,* 747–749.

Stiller, A., Obe, G., Bool, I., & Pribilla, W. (1983). No elevation of the frequencies of chromosomal aberrations as a consequence of handling cytostatic drugs. *Mutation Research, 121,* 253–259.

Stoikes, M. E., Carlson, J. D., Farris, F. F. , & Walker, P. R. (1987). Permeability of latex and polyvinyl chloride gloves to fluorouracil and methotrexate. *American Journal of Hospital Pharmacology, 44,* 1341–1346.

Stucker, I., Hirsch, A., & Doloy, T. (1986). Urine mutagenicity, chromosomal abnormalities and sister chromatid exchanges in lymphocytes of nurses handling cytostatic drugs. *International Archives of Occupational Environmental Health, 57,* 195–205.

Stucker, I., Caillard, J. F., Collin, R., et al. (1990). Risk of spontaneous abortion among nurses handling antineoplastic drugs. *Scandinavian Journal of Work Environment Health, 16,* 102–107.

U.S. Department of Health and Human Services, Public Health Service, National Institutes of Health. (1992). *Recommendations for the safe handling of cytotoxic drugs.* NIH Publication No. 92-2621.

U.S. Department of Health and Human Services, Public Health Service, Centers for Disease Control, National Institute for Occupational Safety and Health. (1988). *Guidelines for protecting the safety and health of health care workers.* DHHS (NIOSH) Publication No. 88-119.

U.S. Department of Labor, Occupational Safety and Health Administration (1984). *Respiratory protection standard.* 29 CFR 1910.134.

U.S. Department of Labor, Occupational Safety and Health Administration (1986). *Work practice guidelines for personnel dealing with cytotoxic (antineoplastic) drugs.* OSHA Publication No. 8-1.1.

U.S. Department of Labor, Occupational Safety and Health Administration (1989). *Hazard communication standard.* 29 CFR 1910.1200, as amended February 9, 1994.

U.S. Department of Labor, Occupational Safety and Health Administration. (1990). *Access to employee and medical records standard.* 29 CFR 1910.20.

U.S. Department of Labor, Occupational Safety and Health Administration. (1991). *Occupational exposure to bloodborne pathogens standard.* 29 CFR 1910.1030.

Vaccari, F. L., Tonat, K., DeChristoforo, R., Gallelli, J. F., & Zimmerman, P. F. (1984). Disposal of antineoplastic wastes at the NIH. *American Journal of Hospital Pharmacology, 41,* 87–92.

Valanis, B., Vollmer, W. M., Labuhn, K., Glass, A., & Corelle, C. (1992). Antineoplastic drug handling protection after OSHA guidelines: Comparison by profession, handling activity, and work site. *Journal of Occupational Medicine, 34,* 149–155.

Venitt, S., Crofton-Sleigh, C., Hunt, J., Speechley, V., & Briggs, K. (1984). Monitoring exposure of nursing and pharmacy personnel to cytotoxic drugs: Urinary mutation assays and urinary platinum as markers of absorption. *Lancet, i,* 74–76.

Waksvik, H., Klepp, O., & Brogger, A. (1981). Chromosome analyses of nurses handling cytostatic agents. *Cancer Treatment Reports, 65,* 607–610.

Wall, R. L., & Clausen, K. P. (1975). Carcinoma of the urinary bladder in patients receiving cyclophosphamide. *New England Journal of Medicine, 293,* 271–273.

Weisburger, J. H., Griswold, D. P., Prejean, J. D., et al. (1975). Tumor induction by cytostatics. The carcinogenic properties of some of the principal drugs used in clinical cancer chemotherapy. *Recent Results Cancer Research, 52,* 1–17.

Zimmerman, P. F., Larsen, R. K., Barkley, E. W., & Gallelli, J. F. (1981). Recommendations for the safe handling of injectable antineoplastic drug products. *American Journal of Hospital Pharmacology, 38,* 1693–1695.